HEALTHY EXPECTATIONS

Preparing a Healthy Body for a Healthy Baby

PAMELA SMITH, R.D.

CREATION HOUSE

HEALTHY EXPECTATIONS by Pamela Smith
Published by Creation House
Strang Communications Company
600 Rinehart Road
Lake Mary, Florida 32746
Web site: http://www.creationhouse.com

All Scripture quotations are from the Holy Bible, New
International Version. Copyright © 1973, 1978, 1984,
International Bible Society. Used by permission.

Typography by Lillian L. McAnally

Library of Congress Cataloging-in-Publication Data

Smith, Pamela M.
    Healthy expectations : preparing a healthy body for a healthy
baby/Pamela Smith
p.   cm.
Includes bibliographical references and index.
ISBN 0-88419-526-0 (hardback)
1. Pregnant women—Health and hygiene.
2. Pregnancy—Nutritional aspects. I. Title.
RG556.S647   1998   98-2909
618.2′4—dc21   CIP

89012345 BVG 87654321

Dedicated to . . .

My precious grandmother, Otha Hensley. Though you have passed on, your ninety-five years on earth were truly a gift that will keep on giving. Your twelve children, thirty-four grandchildren, sixty-seven great-grandchildren, that special great-great-grandson, and those to come "arise and call you blessed"!

My incredible mother, Mae Martin. You didn't just carry me and nourish me through pregnancy, you continued to carry me through my todays with your awesome love and care. Your "healthy expectations" for me are food for my soul—and I am so very grateful to be your daughter.

Acknowledgements to . . .

All those who played tremendously important roles in the conception, growth, and delivery of *Healthy Expectations:*

Carolyn Coats, who co-labored with me to produce the seed for *Healthy Expectations— Perfectly Pregnant.* Your life, your love, and your friendship fuel my writing today.

Tom Freiling, whose vision for this book has now become reality. Thank you for being so open to ideas and so gifted in bringing the good ones into being—you make it fun!

Barb, Lillian, Debbie, and Alyse, whose editorial giftings and talents made this into a "just-about-perfect" baby—and a beautiful one!

Rob, Lindy, Mike, Denise, Ethel, and Leyna, who are anxious and ready to bring *Healthy Expectations* to the world—thank you for your zeal!

My husband, Larry, and daughters Danielle, and Nicole, who so lovingly supported me through the months of waiting—you're awesome and I love you!

Contents

Part 5: New Life—After Baby

List of Charts and Tables

A BABY IS GOD'S OPINION THAT LIFE SHOULD GO ON.

D ear Mom-to-be,
New life has been created inside you, and you have been given a special privilege—the joy of nurturing your baby within until birth! Eating well is a way to express your love for your baby right from the very start. Good nutrition is the gift that only you can give your baby, but that gift goes on—and keeps on—giving! The food you eat is the food that makes your baby healthy, well-nourished, and happy. Such a blessed baby starts life with an advantage that carries on throughout a bright future; every aspect of your baby's life will be affected by nutrition that starts long before birth. No matter what stage of pregnancy you may be in, applying these principles imme- diately will have big payoffs.

I see many of my pregnant patients for the first time just a few weeks before delivery. It is common to hear frustration, maybe a little guilt and fear, that they had not been eating so well throughout the pregnancy.

It is important to displace those negative feelings with the truth that our bodies have been fearfully and wonderfully made. Any pos- itive nutrition change—in any measure, at any time—brings sure rewards, today and tomorrow. If there have been deficiencies in the past few months, the body attempts to cover them and uses the good nutrition now being received to miraculously fill in the gaps.

Yes, it takes a conscious effort to provide your baby with the very best. No maternal instinct draws you to a good diet and keeps you from what is harmful, but the reward of a healthy baby and child is far worth the effort!

You see, you have been created as the perfect host for your baby. You freely give—even without knowing you are—to whatever the need may be. In the first few weeks after conception, a feeding mechanism—the placenta—begins to be formed within your body. Your formed placenta not only delivers food, fluid, and oxygen to your baby, but it also acts as a screen, attempting to block the entry of toxic substances into your baby's bloodstream. Unfortunately, many unwanted substances can still get through to your baby. For this reason, your close focus on what you eat and how you live allows you to serve as the healthy "gatekeeper" to your precious little one.

My goal, and the goal of improved nutrition, is to allow you to be receiving *while* you are truly serving and giving to your baby. The Book of Proverbs tells us that "[s]he who refreshes others will [herself] be refreshed."* This cannot be truer than when you are providing the very best for your baby. You sow—and both the baby and you reap! You will quickly see that once you begin to *eat* well, you will begin to *feel* well. You will see a big difference in your energy level, your stamina, and in your skin, hair, nails, and eyes right away. It works that way because wellness—and beauty—is an inside-out job!

My principles are based on a realistic and positive approach to healthy living and do not rely on theoretical advice that doesn't work in the "real world." My advice is focused toward what *to do*, rather than what *not to do*. I have included special meal plans to guide you through the different stages of your pregnancy, along with recipes and menus to meet your needs and those of your developing child. I have also provided a can't-live-without manual on the "What Abouts . . . " of pregnancy—giving you an understanding of what's occurring, the needs that must be met, and natural remedies to get your body working at its natural best.

If you are not yet pregnant, you will benefit even more from these principles and guidance. You'll know how your diet should be planned, and you'll learn what to expect during your pregnancy. Start using the meal plans and recipes right now to get you on the road to eating right.

The months of pregnancy are some of the most incredible

*Proverbs 11:25

months of a woman's life. From the first moment you receive a definite POSITIVE from the pregnancy test, from the moment the possibility of being pregnant becomes an awesome reality, you are thrust into months of wonder and anticipation. They are a time of preparation for the physical, emotional, and spiritual you. You are not only giving birth to a precious life—you are giving birth to motherhood. Your time of pregnancy is not only the knitting together of the baby, it is a preparation for your glorious new life—a time to build healthy expectations for your body, heart, and soul.

These words are meant to guide and direct, not to make you feel inadequate. Your pregnancy doesn't need to be burdened down with a list of rules and things to feel guilty about—but instead needs loving direction and answers to questions like, "What in the world am I going to do now?"

Let these words and principles lead you through this journey with health, grace, joy, and laughter. Rather than being robbed of the satisfaction and delight of your pregnancy by a tidal wave of morning sickness or fears—learn what you can do to walk in the glory of creation. May these days of wonder be explainable only in terms of God!

—*Pamela Smith, R.D.*

Part 1

BUILDING BLOCKS TO A
HEALTHY BABY

1

EATING WELL, LIVING WELL—PREGNANT!

EACH CHILD IS AN ADVENTURE INTO A BETTER LIFE, AN OPPORTUNITY TO CHANGE THE OLD PATTERN AND MAKE IT NEW.

Burritos, peanut butter chips, Chef Boy-ar-dee ravioli, and Fruit Loops straight from the box—are these the food cravings from a college dorm? Or, maybe, dinnertime fare for an on-the-go person living alone? Nope.

These are foods that babies are often made of—the culinary cravings of many of my very pregnant patients. Although there is a chance that someone, somewhere, craves the stereotypical pickles and ice cream, most of those I counsel enlist my help in the battle between their old food friends and patterns and the necessary eating improvements mandated by their desire for a healthy pregnancy.

Many of my patients are health-conscious eaters, well-educated nutritionally, and committed to smart food choices. We work together to bridge their normal nutritional beliefs and behavior over into their pregnancy for building a healthy baby. By understanding the physiological changes behind pregnancy symptoms and how to manage them, my patients are able to stabilize their eating for the duration of their pregnancy. They are also able to grab hold of an energy level they thought impossible—especially while pregnant!

But not all of my patients are quite so "nutritionally correct." Take Heidi as an example. Heidi had always been naturally thin, the kind of person that others envy. She struggled to keep weight *on* and was used to hearing people say, "You're so lucky—you can eat all the garbage you want!" And garbage she did eat—whenever and whatever she chose.

Heidi's days are familiar to many. She awakens with a blaring alarm and struggles to get up in the morning. She's not hungry for breakfast, and she reports, "Busy people can't take time for that anyway." A diet soda and doughnut midmorning would carry her fine until lunch, and she'd have a quick burger or personal pizza on the run. If Heidi is feeling particularly healthy, she may opt for a big salad and would feel stoic about it, even if she did pour on the dressing. Then, around 3:00 to 3:30 in the afternoon, she would start to look for a candy bar . . . or chips . . . or soda . . . or something, feeling like she just wouldn't make it through the day without it. But her personal arsenic hour would be the beginning of a night filled with nonstop eating—because weight was no problem, Heidi had never considered her eating to be a problem either.

Now, however, eating couldn't be so thoughtless. In a heartbeat (her baby's!), Heidi was needing to jump from a life filled with Twinkies, fries, and hit-and-miss eating, to one that she considered to be monk-like . . . overwhelming . . . and very confusing.

A morning-sick and information-overloaded Heidi sat before me saying, "Pam, consider me nutritionally illiterate. I know there's been a lot of information out there about how to eat right, but I just never bothered with it. Now I'm pregnant, and I *know* that I have to eat better. I'm sick, and I *need* to eat better. I *want* to meet the needs of my baby the best way I can. I just don't have a clue how to do it."

Heidi needed a lot more than counseling; she needed a crash course in nutrition. She knew that new life was being created inside of her, and she had the joy of nurturing her baby to birth. But, there was no maternal instinct that was going to draw her to a good diet and keep her from an unhealthy one—she needed some firm directions.

So, Heidi, and anyone else out there who finds herself pregnant but lost in this new world of nutrition . . . *Healthy Expectations* will lead you into the eat-right prescription—learning to nourish your body with great food for your body, soul, and spirit.

Close your eyes, take a deep breath, and put your hands over your womb. Send heart messages of love and welcome to your baby growing inside. Do this several times a day—rejoicing in the miracle of God.

Healthy Mom, Healthy Baby

Think of pregnancy as a twelve-month experience—a minimum of three months to prepare a healthy body for a healthy baby—and nine months to build a strong baby with food and love. It is also just a beginning—not only is a baby being brought into the world, so is a mother. Be encouraged that the same way of eating that provides optimal health for you is the same kind of eating that keeps your baby healthy, happy, and well-nourished. Your baby can start life with an advantage that carries on throughout a bright future. Every aspect of your baby's life will be affected by nutrition that starts long before birth.

We now have exciting evidence showing that your healthy eating before and during pregnancy not only impacts the growth and development of your little one, but prevents birth defects and impacts your baby's immunity system and chemical balance, even his intelligence, throughout his growing years.

For example, recent studies have shown that babies of proper birth weight have lower levels of triglycerides, higher levels of protective HDL cholesterol, and a lower incidence of heart disease throughout life. Proper birth weight and gestational-age babies also have less insulin resistance, possibly resulting in less susceptibility to diabetes. Another study showed that lower weight gain of the mother between fifteen and thirty-five weeks gestation was related to higher blood pressure when their child was ten to twelve years old.

Possibly the most impacting research in this decade was a landmark study done in several countries showing that proper intake of the B vitamin folacin, or folic acid, in pregnancy can prevent up to 72 percent of such neural tube defects as spina bifida. These dramatic findings have led the United States Public Health Service to recommend that all women of childbearing age who are capable of becoming pregnant consume four hundred micrograms of folic acid each day. Women who have had a child with this kind of neural tube defect are at even higher risk, so are they often advised to supplement with even higher levels, up to eight hundred micrograms each day.

This finding is so important that I encourage my clients who are twenty-something and beyond to supplement with a multivitamin containing this level of folic acid. Not only is there the promise of

4

prevention of these tragic birth defects, there is also evidence that proper folic acid and iron increases a baby's birth weight and length according to its genetic potential.

Much of the same nutrition you learned in fifth grade still applies today, but in your pregnancy, it will be more focused. There are still six essential nutrients—the body's fuel and recipe mix for a healthy life. Every human needs protein, carbohydrates, vitamins, minerals, water, and even fat (in limited amounts); pregnancy only intensifies the need. In order to support the tremendous amount of growth and development that takes place during these special nine months, you will need a diet sufficient in calories and rich in nutrients.

Positively Pregnant!

You may have been waiting for your period to start, but now you are starting to get an idea that you might be pregnant. A pregnancy test is always a good place to begin. Either check with your clinic or physician or purchase a home pregnancy kit. After a positive test, decide on a practitioner and schedule your first prenatal visit.

Selecting a practitioner may be a most difficult task. You need to weigh many considerations as you choose the person who will direct the medical course of your pregnancy and attend the birth of your baby. Before deciding on a practitioner, as you interview your possible choices you should ask about their beliefs: How do they feel about genetic testing? Do they respect your decisions about having it or not? What would they think about your decisions based on the results of such testing? What method of childbirth do they encourage? Will they consult with you and support your desires? Do they routinely do episiotomies? Will they support a home birth if that is an option? Most importantly, do you feel a connection and rapport with this very important person; do you feel a freedom to share what's important to you? These questions and answers will become vital over the course of your pregnancy.

The Best of Times

Pregnancy can be the best of times, yet at times feel like the worst. There is much that you can do to take charge of the experience—and make it simply the most positive time possible. The factors that contribute to a positive experience include:

1. *Your general health.* Being in good overall physical condition gives you the best shot at having a comfortable, vitality-filled pregnancy. Ideally, get chronic conditions like allergies, asthma, diabetes, or back conditions at their stable best before conception. Clear up lingering infections such as urinary tract or yeast infections. Once you become pregnant, continue to take *great* care of you!

2. *Your eating plan.* Following my Healthy Expectations Meal Plan gives you the best chance for a terrific pregnancy. Not only can it better your chances of avoiding or decreasing the miseries of morning sickness and heartburn, it also can help fight excessive fatigue, combat constipation and hemorrhoids, prevent constant bladder infections and anemia, and get you over the hurdle of leg cramps. Not only are you impacting your well-being and enjoyment of this amazing time, but you are also giving your baby the best gift of all—contributing to that sweet one's developing well and being born healthy.

3. *Proper weight gain.* Gaining weight at a steady rate and keeping the gain within the recommended levels (twenty-five to thirty-five pounds) can greatly improve your odds of escaping or minimizing such misery factors as hemorrhoids, varicose veins, stretch marks, backaches, fatigue, heartburn, and shortness of breath. The Healthy Expectations Meal Plan on pages 82–85 will allow you to gain a healthy weight naturally.

4. *Fitness.* Getting enough of the right kind of exercise can help improve your overall well-being. Exercise is important at any time, but especially in repeat pregnancies; abdominal muscles tend to be laxer, making you more susceptible to lots of aches and pains.

5. *The pace of your life.* Living life in the frenzied lane can greatly aggravate—or even cause—many of the most horrific pregnancy symptoms such as morning sickness,

heartburn, fatigue, and backaches. These symptoms are magnified when there are other children to care for in addition to the general cares of life.

Building a Strong Baby With Food and Love

The typical person living life in the fast lane subsists on a diet that is high in fat, sodium, and sugar, and generally low in protein, calcium, and vitamins A and C. This is *not* the recipe for a healthy pregnancy. The key is to replace erratic, sporadic eating with a better-timed routine of smaller meals and smart snacks, more evenly spaced throughout the day. This allows better exposure and use of nutrients, as well as better energy and overall well-being.

Good health habits have never been more imprtant than they are right now. If you are the type of person who already eats well-balanced meals, exercises moderately, gets sufficient rest, and doesn't drink alcohol, smoke, or take drugs, stay the course. If you need an excuse to finally take better care of yourself, let the baby be that excuse. Any positive change at any time during the pregnancy benefits both you and baby—for now and forevermore!

Of course, you aren't the only one with healthy expectations—there's a daddy-in-waiting as well. And now it's time to pass this book on to him . . . the next chapter is written for him and to him. You can sneak a peek if you must and ask him questions about what he will read in the next chapter. Give him the space to grow into the incredible dad he's been created to be. He too will grow strong with food and love.

YOU WILL NEED APPROXIMATELY THREE HUNDRED EXTRA CALORIES PER DAY WHILE YOU ARE PREGNANT. YOU MAY NEED A LITTLE LESS IN THE FIRST TRIMESTER AND A LITTLE MORE IN THE LAST. BUT YOUR VITAMIN AND MINERAL NEEDS JUMP AS MUCH AS 25 TO 100 PERCENT. (SEE THE TABLE OF NUTRIENT SOURCES ON THE NEXT PAGE.) THOSE FEW EXTRA CALORIES DON'T REALLY AMOUNT TO THAT MUCH FOOD. (YOU CAN GET THAT MANY CALORIES IN A LARGE ORDER OF FRIES!) TO GET WHAT IS NEEDED, YOU MUST CAREFULLY CHOOSE WHAT YOU EAT, PACKING IN THE HIGHER AMOUNTS OF VITAMINS, MINERALS, AND PROTEIN.

HEALTHY EXPECTATIONS

Nutrient	Need for	Best Sources
Calcium 1300 mg	Baby's bone development; your bone strength; may keep blood pressure stable; helps to prevent muscle cramps	Milk, cheese, yogurt, dark green leafy veggies, salmon, dried beans
Copper 1.5-3 mg	Preventing anemia; forming baby's bones and nerve fibers	Dried beans, seafood, whole grains, nuts, seeds, raisins
Folic acid 400 mcg	Help in preventing neural tube defects and cleft palate; building strong red blood cell and cell turnover; helps to utilize proteins	Dark green leafy veggies, oranges, strawberries, whole grains, dried beans
Iron 30 mg	Preventing anemia; help baby's weight gain; helps to prevent premature delivery	Lean red meat, fish, seafood, poultry, whole grains, dried fruits, green leafy veggies
Magnesium 320 mg	Bone and tissue building; muscle contractions; nerve transmissions; immune function	Whole grains, wheat germ, beans, dark green veggies, seafood
Protein 75-100 grams	Building baby's cells and tissues; achieving full growth potential	Dairy, meat, fish, poultry, dried beans, peanuts
Riboflavin 1.6 mg	Preventing anemia; builds baby's cells and tissues; helps to utilize energy nutrients	Dairy, eggs, whole grains, dark green leafies, asparagus, seafood, meats, whole grains
Selenium 65 mcg (while pregnant) 75 mcg (while breast-feeding)	Protecting body from free radicals; helps to reduce cancer risk	Brazil nuts, whole grains, seafoods, meat
Vitamin B_6 2.2 mg	Helps to utilize protein; helps in cell turnover and production	Whole grains, eggs, meats, dried beans, nuts, bananas, avocado
Vitamin C 70 mg	Preventing anemia; building strong bones and teeth	Citrus, broccoli, mangoes, red peppers, strawberries
Vitamin B_{12} 2.2 mg	Preventing anemia	Animal products: dairy, meat, eggs
Zinc 15 mg	Cell division; aids proper growth; prevents premature delivery; achieves muscle strength; endurance; healing	Meat, seafood, whole grains, dried beans, nuts, beets, carrots, cabbage

2

A Note to Dad

THE MOST IMPORTANT THING A FATHER CAN DO FOR
HIS CHILDREN IS TO LOVE THEIR MOTHER.

From the moment a woman finds out that she is pregnant, the advice comes pouring in: Eat this. Don't drink that. Do Kegels. Nap. Relax.

But what about you? Here you are, a genuine dad-to-be, and no one is giving you a bit of advice. Yet you have a lot of changing to do as well. The problem is, you don't have all the physical changes of your own body to obsess on, so you have nothing to get your mind off the worries: *Will I be a good father? Can we do this financially? Will the house always look like this? Is this the end of fun forever?* And it's hard to go public with those fears because, well, it just doesn't seem like a "guy thing."

Don't be surprised if your woman is so involved with her own emotions, thoughts, and worries that she has little time or interest in you—or you might be coping with the pregnancy.

Don't be surprised if your concerns come out "sideways" and you find yourself feeling a lot of the same physical symptoms as your wife. Cravings, weight gain, and even morning sickness are all pretty common in dads-to-be! For that reason, get very involved with this pregnancy. And stay involved—go to checkups, ask questions, and read books like this one. As a matter of fact, now that you have this book in your hands, continue reading—right along with Mom. The healthy lifestyle principles employed to nourish your unborn child can become the framework for your new family's healthy life. Encourage your wife to talk to you about her fears and concerns, and, painful as it is, talk about yours. Most importantly, here is some lifesaving advice on how to be absolutely perfect in your vital role in this blessed event:

1. *Do not, under any circumstances, make beeping noises when your very pregnant wife steps backward.* Don't ever let the word *whale* be used in your conversations.

2. *Mention how wonderful your wife looks pregnant . . .* that you never realized how captivating a pregnant woman is, that you are so bored by women who aren't pregnant.

3. *Rave about the exciting and healthy ways you are eating together and how much you love exercising together.* If you find her demanding ice cream with fudge sauce one night, don't mention the fat grams that she counted off to you the day before.

4. *Be a wellspring of sympathy.* Listen to all of your wife's complaints about her body and show your undivided interest.

5. *Frequently discuss how excited you are to be a part of the labor team.* Don't talk about videotaping the delivery very often.

6. *When the grouchies overtake your wife, be amazed that she stays in such a great mood most of the time.* Who wouldn't be a little cranky with all the changes she's going through? Never, never compare her irritability to her past experience with PMS.

7. *Insist that she take a nap while you cook and clean the house,* or pay someone to clean while you go get takeout.

8. *Read books on foot massage and talk about how enjoyable it is to give a foot massage to her.*

The perfect dad-to-be realizes that his most precious gift to the mother of his child is to make her feel loved. With the baby's arrival will come labor you can really share.

3

Building Block 1: Eat Early

WE ALWAYS HAVE TIME FOR THE THINGS WE PUT FIRST.

Although it may not seem like new news, breakfast still is the most important meal of your day—don't leave home without it! If you want to start your day with a boundless energy level, your metabolism in high gear, and proteins actively building you and your baby's new cells, then never skip breakfast!

Build With Breakfast

Breakfast is important to "break the fast" your body has been in during the hours of night rest. Think of your body as a campfire that dies down during the night. In the morning it needs to be stoked up with wood to begin burning vigorously again. Without stoking, the fire will die down with no flames or sparks. Your body is very similar—it awakens in a slowed, fasting state and needs breakfast to rev the body into high gear, allowing better nutrient utilization for you and baby.

Studies show that one out of four women between the ages of twenty-five and thirty-four skip breakfast. With these years being the primary childbearing years, it means that some help is needed on the breakfast front!

If you choose not to eat breakfast, the body not only stays slowed down, but, as in the case of a campfire, the metabolism will die down even more, conserving itself for functioning in this disabled,

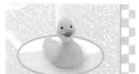

EAT BREAKFAST SOON AFTER YOU GET UP (WITHIN THE FIRST HALF-HOUR OF ARISING). GO LIGHT AND EASY IF TIME IS A PUSH; TRY SOME EAT-AND-GO MEALS LIKE FRESH FRUIT AND SKIM-MILK SHAKES, CHEESE MELTED ON WHOLE-WHEAT TOAST AND FRUIT, OR FRESHLY FRUITED YOGURT WITH A HOMEMADE MUFFIN OR CEREAL. OR TRY THE BREAKFAST RECIPES ON PAGES III–II9.

DON'T LIKE BREAK-FAST FOODS? START YOUR DAY WITH A TURKEY SANDWICH OR A PIECE OF CHEESE PIZZA! THE KEY IS TO HAVE BREAKFAST, HAVE IT SOON, AND HAVE IT BALANCED. THE MEAL DOESN'T HAVE TO BE TRADI-TIONAL—THE BEST THING FOR BREAKFAST IS WHAT YOU WILL EAT.

starved state. Continuing to starve the body will cause it to drag through the day in a slowed-down metabolic state, unable to work efficiently for you and your baby. When the evening "gorge" begins, much of the food will be wasted or stored as fat. All that food can't possibly be used up, because the body isn't burning energy at a fast rate—the fire has already gone out. The food that comes in is like dumping an armful of firewood on a dead fire!

Breakfast also serves to lift ailing blood sugars, which give better energy, and neutralizes gastric acids to help in fighting morning queasiness. It is a vital tool for fighting nausea, so don't ever make the mistake of skipping breakfast because you are queasy—it will only make it worse.

Don't think for a minute that you are cutting calories by skipping breakfast or your healthy snacks; those calories would be burned by the higher metabolic rate. You are only starving your body and your baby of valuable carbohydrates that burn to give you energy and proteins that build your sweet baby.

But Breakfast Makes Me Hungry!

A common reason for skipping breakfast is that it seems to start a voracious appetite machine—making you hungry every few hours. It's true—and it's a good thing! It's all about your body working correctly. When you starve your body in the morning, waste products are released into your system, temporarily depressing your appetite and allowing you to starve without feeling hungry for many hours. Unfortunately, these unhealthy prod-ucts are absorbed by the baby. In addition, you've let your body go into a slowed metabolic state, and you're setting yourself up for a gorge. As soon as you begin to eat, your appetite is really turned on! Not only will you overeat because your blood sugar level has fallen so low, but, like the campfire, your body will not be able to burn those calories well.

If you are feeling queasy and unable to face breakfast, look at the Healthy Expectations Meal Plan on page 82 for help in overcoming morning sickness. This proven meal plan not only includes breakfast, but relies on it for getting the body's chemistries stabilized.

Have three different foods for breakfast—a quick, energy-starting simple carbohydrate (fruit or "soft" juice), a long-lasting complex carbohydrate (grains, cereal, bread, or muffins) and a power-building protein (dairy, eggs, or meats).

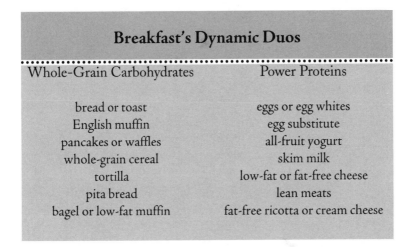

Breakfast's Dynamic Duos

Whole-Grain Carbohydrates	Power Proteins
bread or toast	eggs or egg whites
English muffin	egg substitute
pancakes or waffles	all-fruit yogurt
whole-grain cereal	skim milk
tortilla	low-fat or fat-free cheese
pita bread	lean meats
bagel or low-fat muffin	fat-free ricotta or cream cheese

ACTION STEP 1: EAT BREAKFAST EVERY DAY, STARTING TOMORROW MORNING! USING THE FOLLOWING SAMPLE FOOD DIARY AS A GUIDE, FILL IN A BLANK FOOD DIARY WITH YOUR SUNNY START TO A GREAT DAY!

Sample Breakfast Diary

Your name _Lynn_____   Week beginning _January 15_____

	BREAKFAST	LUNCH	DINNER	COMMENTS & EXERCISE
MONDAY	TIME: 6:30 A.M. 2 SLICES WHOLE-WHEAT TOAST 2 OZ. PART-SKIM MOZZARELLA (MELTED ON TOAST) 1 NECTARINE COFFEE WITH 1% MILK SNACK:	TIME: SNACK:	TIME: SNACK:	COMMITTED!
TUESDAY	TIME: 6:40 A.M. 1fi CUPS NUTRI-GRAIN ALMOND RAISIN CEREAL 1 CUP 1% MILK / CUP HIGH-CALCIUM COTTAGE CHEESE WITH STRAW- SNACK:	TIME: SNACK:	TIME: SNACK:	TIRED
WEDNESDAY	TIME: 6:35 A.M. 1 WHOLE-WHEAT ENGLISH MUFFIN WITH 1 TSP. ALL-FRUIT JAM 2-EGG WHITE OMELET 6 OZ. ORANGE JUICE SNACK:	TIME: SNACK:	TIME: SNACK:	A LITTLE HUNGRY

Building Block 1: Eat Early

Your name _____   Week beginning _____

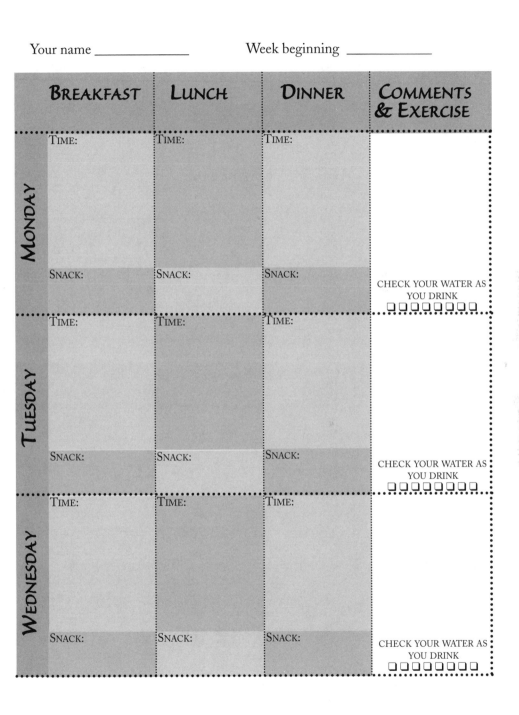

	BREAKFAST	LUNCH	DINNER	COMMENTS & EXERCISE
MONDAY	TIME: SNACK:	TIME: SNACK:	TIME: SNACK:	 CHECK YOUR WATER AS YOU DRINK ▢▢▢▢▢▢▢▢
TUESDAY	TIME: SNACK:	TIME: SNACK:	TIME: SNACK:	 CHECK YOUR WATER AS YOU DRINK ▢▢▢▢▢▢▢▢
WEDNESDAY	TIME: SNACK:	TIME: SNACK:	TIME: SNACK:	 CHECK YOUR WATER AS YOU DRINK ▢▢▢▢▢▢▢▢

HEALTHY EXPECTATIONS

Your name _____   Week beginning _____

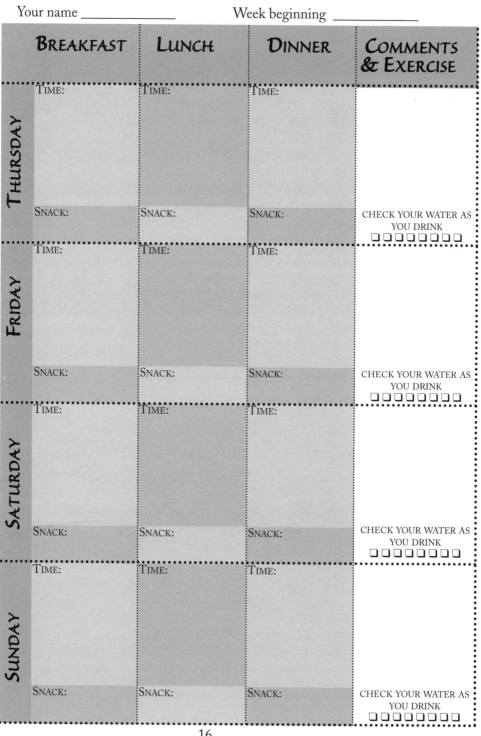

	BREAKFAST	LUNCH	DINNER	COMMENTS & EXERCISE
THURSDAY	TIME: SNACK:	TIME: SNACK:	TIME: SNACK:	 CHECK YOUR WATER AS YOU DRINK ☐☐☐☐☐☐☐
FRIDAY	TIME: SNACK:	TIME: SNACK:	TIME: SNACK:	 CHECK YOUR WATER AS YOU DRINK ☐☐☐☐☐☐☐
SATURDAY	TIME: SNACK:	TIME: SNACK:	TIME: SNACK:	 CHECK YOUR WATER AS YOU DRINK ☐☐☐☐☐☐☐
SUNDAY	TIME: SNACK:	TIME: SNACK:	TIME: SNACK:	 CHECK YOUR WATER AS YOU DRINK ☐☐☐☐☐☐☐

Building Block 2: Eat Often

TRAIN UP A CHILD IN THE WAY HE SHOULD GO—AND
WALK THERE YOURSELF.

Once you get your day started with breakfast, continue to eat "minimeals" often throughout the day, about every two to two-and-one-half hours. Remember the campfire story? Healthy and wise snacking is like throwing wood on a fire all throughout the day to keep it burning well. It will result in more energy, a healthy, proper weight gain, and will provide a constant source of nutrients in your bloodstream to be carried to the placenta and your baby. By keeping your body supplied with the right things at the right time, you will better prevent nausea and fatigue. Not eating evenly throughout the day can leave you weak and dizzy, with an appetite raging out of control.

Try to eat consistently and evenly each day, including three meals with at least two healthy snacks. Ideally, you should eat 25 percent of your calories at breakfast, 25 percent at lunch, 25 percent at dinner, and the other 25 percent in healthy snacks. The Healthy Expectations Meal Plan is designed to provide you with this wise pattern of eating.

Power Snacking Smarts

When most people think of snacks, they picture potato chips, candy, and sodas. These types of snacks are "empty calories," providing high amounts of fats, sugars, salt, and calories but little or no vitamins or minerals.

A healthy snack provides you with needed nutrition and will keep your blood sugar level from dropping too low, leaving you sleepy and craving sweets. It will keep your metabolism burning high, with your and your baby's needs satisfied, and still not load you down with unwanted, unneeded fat, salt, sugar, and calories.

Make snacks into power combos of energy-giving carbohydrates and power proteins. Keep power snacks available wherever you are—in your car, your desk drawer, your briefcase, a purse, or a diaper bag! They can be as simple as fresh fruit or a box of raisins with low-fat cheese or yogurt, a half sandwich, or even a trail mixture of dry-roasted peanuts, sunflower seeds, and dried fruit. When you don't have good choices available, you're likely to reach for an unhealthy snack or eat nothing at all. Neither are healthy or happy options!

No refrigeration? Keep these foods available for grab-and-go snacking:

Complex Carbohydrates
Whole-wheat bread or pita rounds, rice cakes or Wasa bread, Harvest Crisps crackers, Guiltless Gourmet No-Oil Tortilla Chips, Baked Tostitos, whole-grain cereals *(Shredded Wheat, Müesli, Nutri-Grain, Raisin Squares)*

Proteins
Laughing Cow Light cheese *(doesn't need refrigeration)*, Parmalet skim or 1% milk in boxes *(also no refrigeration)*, natural peanut butter, Trail Mix *(pg. 19)*, pop-top cans of tuna *(water-packed)* and chicken, fat-free bean dips

Simple Carbohydrates
Small boxes of raisins, dried apricots, boxes of unsweetened juices

ACTION STEP 2: PLAN YOUR DAY TO INCLUDE POWER SNACKS AND MEALS TO FUEL YOUR BABY AND YOU EVERY TWO TO TWO-AND-ONE-HALF HOURS THROUGHOUT YOUR DAY. CHOOSE FROM ANY OF THE POWER SNACK SUGGESTIONS, OR CREATIVELY PUT TOGETHER YOUR OWN. FILL IN A FOOD DIARY WITH THE POWER SNACKS YOU HAVE EACH DAY. (MAKE COPIES OF THE FOOD DIARY ON PAGES 15–16 TO USE.) IT MAY LOOK SOMETHING LIKE THE POWER SNACKING SAMPLE DIARY ON PAGE 20.

The following table gives some power snack suggestions that balance carbohydrate with protein:

POWER SNACK CHOICES

Baked Tostitos or Guiltless Gourmet tortilla chips with $^1/_3$ cup fat-free bean dip and salsa

$^1/_2$ sandwich on whole-grain kaiser roll or whole-wheat bread, made with turkey and mozzarella (with light mayo and touch of mustard) or ham and fat-free cheese (with light mayo and touch of mustard)

$^1/_2$ cinnamon raisin bagel with light cream cheese and all-fruit spread

Whole-grain cereal with skim milk

Fat-Free Philadelphia Cheese Spread and whole-grain crackers

Charlie's Lunch Kit or small pop-top can of tuna with whole-grain crackers

Harvest Crisps crackers or Raisin Squares cereal with Laughing Cow Light cheese wedge or low-fat string cheese

Health Valley graham crackers or Quaker Banana Nut rice cakes with 2 Tbsp. natural peanut butter

Crispbread crackers with sliced turkey and Dijon mustard

Light popcorn with 2 Tbsp. freshly grated Parmesan cheese

Stonyfield Farm yogurt or plain, nonfat yogurt mixed with all-fruit spread

12 grapes or 10 fresh strawberries with low-fat string cheese or Armenian cheese

1 cup of gazpacho with low-fat string cheese

Fruit shake (skim milk blended with frozen fruit and vanilla extract)

Low-fat cheese tortellini salad in vinaigrette with carrots and celery

Dill tortilla rolls: tortilla with fat-free cream cheese, lemon juice, fresh dill, and creole seasoning

Trail Mix (1 cup unsalted, dry-roasted peanuts; 1 cup unsalted, dry-roasted, shelled sunflower seeds; and 2 cups raisins)—make in abundance and bag into $^1/_4$-cup portions

Homemade low-fat bran muffin and skim milk

HEALTHY EXPECTATIONS

Power Snacking Sample Diary

Your name *Lynn*   Week beginning *March 22*

	BREAKFAST	LUNCH	DINNER	COMMENTS & EXERCISE
MONDAY	TIME: 6:30 A.M. BAGEL WITH 2 TBSP. PEANUT BUTTER 8 OZ. SKIM MILK SMALL BANANA	TIME: 11:45 A.M. TUNA SANDWICH ON WHOLE-WHEAT BREAD APPLE CAFFEINE-FREE DIET PEPSI	TIME: 5:30 P.M. SPAGHETTI WITH MEAT SAUCE SLICED ZUCCHINI SALAD WITH ITALIAN DRESSING WATER	9:00 A.M. – HUNGRY 3:00 P.M. – FEEL GOOD 6:30 P.M. – WALKED; HAD ENERGY 8:30 P.M. – HUNGRY
	SNACK: 8 OZ. STRAWBERRY YOGURT	SNACK: 1 SLICE BREAD 2 OZ. TURKEY WITH MUSTARD	SNACK: 1 CUP RAISIN SQUARES 1 CUP MILK	CHECK YOUR WATER AS YOU DRINK ☑☑☑☑☑☑☑☑
TUESDAY	TIME:	TIME:	TIME:	
	SNACK:	SNACK:	SNACK:	CHECK YOUR WATER AS YOU DRINK ☐☐☐☐☐☐☐☐
WEDNESDAY	TIME:	TIME:	TIME:	
	SNACK:	SNACK:	SNACK:	CHECK YOUR WATER AS YOU DRINK ☐☐☐☐☐☐☐☐

5

BUILDING BLOCK 3:
EAT BALANCED

LOVE IS LIKE THE FIVE LOAVES AND TWO FISHES—IT
DOESN'T START TO MULTIPLY UNTIL YOU GIVE IT AWAY.

Balance is vital to utilizing nutrients optimally. And balance is more than just a pretty plate—it's getting the right foods at the right time—always including carbohydrates and proteins at every meal and snack.

These two nutrients have different yet equally vital functions. Carbohydrates are 100 percent pure energy! They are your body's fuel, designed to burn fast, clean, and pure. Carbohydrates should be eaten with a protein to protect the protein from being wasted as a less efficient source of energy. This allows protein to be used for its most important functions: as building blocks for you and your baby. The proteins you eat build new cells in you and your baby, boost your metabolism, build body muscle, as well as provide for growth of the placenta and uterus. Pregnant moms who eat sufficient protein are more apt to have babies who have achieved their proper birth length according to their full genetic potential. Proteins keep the body fluids in balance, they heal and fight infections, and they make beautiful skin, hair, and nails. Always remember—carbohydrates burn and proteins build!

Energy-Giving Carbohydrates

Carbohydrates are found in plant foods (wheat, corn, oats, rice, barley, fruits, and vegetables) and are nutritional heavyweights themselves. They are packed with fibers, vitamins, and minerals that allow your body to stay operative from a point of strength. Again, carbohydrate is 100 percent energy for your body and baby.

Some forms of carbohydrates are digested and absorbed quite simply, allowing them to be quick-burning forms of energy. These are called simple carbohydrates and are found in fruits and crunchy vegetables. Others require more time to get into a usable form of energy; they are digested more slowly and are absorbed evenly into the system as fuel. These are called the complex carbohydrates. This form of energy is found in grains, root vegetables, and legumes.

Carbohydrate-containing foods and the nutrients they contain are essential to your baby's growth and development. Whole grain carbohydrates are particularly valuable because they have not had the outer layers of grain removed—they contain many more vitamins, minerals, and fiber than the refined, white products (even though possibly enriched). In addition, whole-grain carbohydrates are rich in the B vitamins, which are particularly crucial for the growth of your baby's cells, organ and limb formation, efficient digestion, metabolism of foods in you, and the prevention of anemia and possibly toxemia. (Read more about anemia and toxemia on pages 56 and 194.)

Vitamin B_6, found in whole-grain carbohydrates, is especially crucial in pregnancy—it is thought to be a major deterrent to nausea and fatigue and appears to play a role in the prevention of toxemia. Folic acid is now known to be crucial for preventing neural tube birth defects such as spina bifida. It is *so* important that most physicians recommend that their patients supplement their diet with four hundred micrograms of folic acid for the three months before conception and throughout pregnancy.

You need at least six servings of whole-grain carbohydrate foods each day. And always remember to balance them with lots of low-fat power proteins!

ENERGY-GIVING CARBOHYDRATES

Simple Carbohydrates
(Fruits and Nonstarchy Vegetables)

All fruits and fruit juices

apples, apricots, bananas, berries, cherries, dates, grapefruit, grapes, kiwis, lemons, limes, melons, nectarines, oranges, peaches, pears, pineapples, plums, raisins

(Generally one serving of simple carbohydrate is obtained from $1/2$ cup fruit, $1/2$ cup fruit juice, or $1/8$ cup dried fruit. This gives 10 grams of simple carbohydrate.)

Nonstarchy vegetables

asparagus, beets, broccoli, Brussels sprouts, cabbage, carrots, cauliflower, celery, green beans, green leafy vegetables, kale, mushrooms, okra, onions, snow peas, sugar snap peas, summer squash, tomatoes, zucchini

(Generally one serving of simple carbohydrate is obtained from $1/2$ cup cooked vegetables or 1 cup raw vegetables or juice. This gives 10 grams of simple carbohydrate.)

Complex Carbohydrates
(Grains and Starchy Vegetables)

Grains

The following amounts provide one serving of complex carbohydrate, giving 15 grams:

barley, bulgur, couscous, grits, kasha, millet, or polenta, cooked . . . . $1/2$ cup
bread . . . . .1 slice
cereals . . . . .1 oz.
($1/4$ cup of a concentrated cereal such as Grape-Nuts or granola, $1/2$ to $3/4$ cup flaked cereals, and 1 cup puffed cereals)
crackers or mini-rice cakes 5
crispbread or rice cakes 2
oats, uncooked . . . . $1/3$ cup
pasta or rice, cooked . . . . . $1/2$ cup
fat-free tortillas
(flour or corn) 1
wheat germ . . . . $1/4$ cup

Starchy vegetables

black-eyed peas, corn, green peas, lima beans, parsnips, potatoes (white and sweet), rutabagas, turnips, winter squash

(Generally one serving of complex carbohydrate is obtained from $1/2$ cup cooked starchy vegetables, giving 15 grams.)

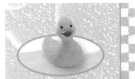

YOUR NEED FOR PRO-
TEIN INCREASES
GREATLY DURING
PREGNANCY—
I RECOMMEND UP TO
ONE HUNDRED GRAMS
OF PROTEIN EACH
DAY, ESPECIALLY FOR
HIGHER-RISK
PREGNANCIES.
SPECIFICALLY, THIS IS
1.5 GRAMS PER KILO-
GRAMS (2.2 POUNDS)
OF YOUR BODY
WEIGHT.

NEVER, NEVER
BELIEVE ANYBODY OR
ANYTHING THAT
TELLS YOU THAT YOU
DON'T NEED PROTEIN
OR TO EAT IT ONLY
ONCE A DAY. YOU ARE
ROBBING YOUR BODY
AND BABY OF PRO-
TEIN'S HEALING AND
BUILDING POWER ALL
DAY LONG.

Refining and Enriching: A Robbery That's Legal!

Consider this story: A man walking down the street was approached by a robber who, at gunpoint, forced the man to turn over his valuables, including all that he was wearing. After the man stripped, the thief said, "I have just refined you!" Then he returned only four items: the man's watch, one shoe, his undershirt, and his necktie. The thief proclaimed, "I have just enriched you!"

Returning four nutrients and leaving out twenty-one is what this enrichment caper is all about. When a whole-wheat berry is refined, every nutrient is affected (twenty-one are completely lost), and all of its protective fiber is stripped away. In the enrichment process, only four are added back.

Don't be fooled by advertisements! White, refined carbohydrates, even though enriched, are never as good nutritionally as whole grains.

Power Proteins

Your need for protein increases greatly during pregnancy. It is the "new you," and it becomes a building block for you and your baby's new cells. The brain cell development of your baby depends on your protein intake—as does the growth of the uterus and placenta. Research has shown that inadequate protein intake in pregnancy, like inadequate calories, can result in babies that are smaller than normal at birth.

Protein boosts your metabolism, builds body muscles and nerve tissue, as well as provides for growth of the placenta and uterus. It serves to keep body fluids in balance (excessive swelling and fluid retention is often caused by inadequate protein) and makes beautiful hair, skin, and nails for your baby. Protein works to replace worn-out cells and to regulate your body functions.

The diets of our time have promised protein to be the food to eat for weight loss. The truth is that an all-protein, no-carbohydrate diet so imbalances the body that you do lose weight. It's just the wrong kind of weight loss—mostly water and muscle mass, and little fat. Remember this after delivery as you are eating to return to your best shape. And keep in mind right now that the protein and carbohydrates you eat are the fuels on which your body runs and your baby grows.

What Is Protein, and Where Do I Find It?

Anything that comes from an animal (poultry, fish, meat, eggs, cheese, milk, and yogurt) gives you complete protein, supplying all the essential amino acids that your body can't make or store. (See the table of Power Proteins on page 26.)

The only plant source of quality protein, a miraculous one, is the legume family (dried beans and peanuts)—their pods absorb nitrogen from the soil and become an excellent high-fiber, low-fat protein source. Yet, because they lack sufficient amounts of one or more of the essential amino acids, they are considered "incomplete" proteins. They must be eaten with a grain (corn, wheat, rice, or oat products) or a seed (sunflower, sesame, pumpkin) to be complete. Examples of high-quality dynamic duos are: peanut butter on bread, black beans over rice, beans and tortillas or cornbread, or a peanut and sunflower seed Trail Mix. Generally, $^1/_2$ cup of cooked beans serves as two ounces protein when mixed with an appropriate grain or seed, and $^3/_4$ cup equals three ounces protein.

Women need at least seventy grams of protein a day during pregnancy, and I recommend up to one hundred grams for most of my patients. Generally, one ounce of meat contains about seven grams of protein, meaning you need a minimum of ten to thirteen ounces per day. This may sound like a lot, but in reality this need can be met by eating three ounces of protein at meals and two ounces at each power snack.

It's important for you to know that the amount of protein eaten is not the only secret to a healthy pregnancy. Equally important is the need to take in protein in smaller, evenly distributed amounts every two to two-and-one-half hours. Protein is not stored, so it must be replenished frequently throughout the day, each and every day of your pregnancy. It also needs to eaten with lots of energy-giving carbohydrates to protect the protein from being wasted as a less-efficient source of energy.

While pregnant, your snack should include at least two ounces protein, and your meals should provide three to four ounces after cooking. If possible, get a food scale and periodically weigh your protein portion to be sure you are getting enough. Getting enough protein at the right time is a vital ingredient for making a healthy mom and baby.

POWER PROTEINS

Each serving equals 1 ounce of protein (7 grams)

- 4 oz. nonfat milk or nonfat plain yogurt
- 1 oz. (or $\frac{1}{4}$ cup grated) low-fat cheeses
- $\frac{1}{4}$ cup 1 percent low-fat or nonfat cottage cheese or part-skim or fat-free ricotta
- 1 egg (particularly use egg whites)
- 1 oz. fish (or $\frac{1}{4}$ cup flaked fish)
- $\frac{1}{4}$ cup seafood (crab, lobster)
- 5 seafood (clams, shrimp, oysters, or scallops)
- 1 oz. (or $\frac{1}{4}$ cup chopped) turkey, Cornish hens
- 1 oz. chicken (or $\frac{1}{4}$ cup chopped)
- 1 oz. beef, pork, lamb, veal (lean, trimmed)
- $\frac{1}{4}$ cup legumes (black beans, garbanzo beans, Great Northern beans, kidney beans, lentils, navy beans, peanuts, red beans, split peas, soybeans, and soy products such as tofu and soy milk)
   Although a plant food, legumes contain valuable protein if eaten with a grain—corn, wheat, rice, oats—or a seed—pumpkin, sunflower, sesame.
- 2 Tbsp. natural peanut butter

Choose your food choices wisely—make them low-fat. One of the drawbacks of eating more protein is that many popular proteins are high in fat. Fat, although an essential nutrient and needed in small amounts, is also the major dietary risk factor in many killer diseases.

By choosing the low-fat versions of protein foods, you will get all of their goodness (protein builders, calcium, magnesium, iron, and zinc) without the risk. A particularly wise choice for low-fat proteins while pregnant is fish—an excellent source of omega-3 fatty acids. These good-for-you oils have been shown to protect the heart, ease rheumatoid arthritis pain—and even improve infants' IQs. (Good news: Omega-3s are also found in breast milk!) Omega-3s may also reduce the chances of premature birth and low birth weight. In addition, one type of omega-3 known as docosahexaenoic acid, or DHA, is important for development of the brain and retina.

Unborn babies totally rely on Mom for their supply of DHA, accumulating most of it during the last trimester of pregnancy. Some women are so drained of their stores of this omega-3 that researchers have begun to speculate that their low stores may contribute to postpartum depression. We've heard that fish is brain food—but is it good "mood food" as well?

Because fish-oil supplements are not deemed safe or effective for pregnant women, the simplest and best way to build up stores of omega-3s is to eat more fish, ideally two to three three-ounce servings of cooked fish per week. All fish contain these healthy fatty acids—salmon, tuna, mackerel, and shellfish are the richest sources. Swordfish also is a good source, but the FDA advises pregnant women to limit their intake of both swordfish and shark because they also contain higher levels of methyl mercury than other fish. This toxic compound can cause neurological damage to your baby—so stay clear of them, or have no more than a three-ounce serving once a month. My advice—considering there are so many other great choices of healthy fish—*when in doubt, leave it out!*

ACTION STEP 3: CONTINUE KEEPING TRACK OF WHAT YOU EAT, WHEN YOU EAT, AND HOW YOU FEEL. CHECK YOUR CHOICES FOR EACH POWER SNACK AND MEAL TO ASSURE THAT YOU ARE GETTING A BALANCE OF WHOLE CARBOHYDRATES AND LOW-FAT PROTEINS. THIS IS THE VERY BEST WAY TO MEET YOUR NEEDS AND YOUR BABY'S! YOUR DIARY MAY LOOK SOMETHING LIKE THE SAMPLE ON PAGE 28.

Sample Food Diary

Your name *Lynn*   Week beginning *February 2*

	BREAKFAST	LUNCH	DINNER	COMMENTS & EXERCISE
FRIDAY	PROTEIN: 6:35 A.M. 2 EGGS COMPLEX CARB: 2 SLICES WHOLE-WHEAT TOAST SIMPLE CARB: 1 ORANGE ADDED FAT: SNACK*: 6 CRACKERS; 2 STRING	PROTEIN: 11:30 A.M. 1 CHICKEN BREAST COMPLEX CARB: 1 LARGE BAKED POTATO SIMPLE CARB: 1 SIDE VEGETABLE AND DISH OF STRAWBERRIES ADDED FAT: 1 TBSP. SOUR CREAM SNACK*: HALF A TURKEY SANDWICH;	PROTEIN: 7:00 P.M. SALMON STEAK COMPLEX CARB: WILD RICE SIMPLE CARB: BROCCOLI; MIXED GREEN SALAD ADDED FAT: SALAD DRESSING SNACK*: CEREAL AND MILK	UP AT 5:45 A.M.—6 OZ. APPLE JUICE; WALKED 40 MINUTES 4:00 P.M.—GETTING TIRED 4:45 P.M.—FEEL BETTER AFTER SNACK 9:30 P.M.—NOT HUNGRY; STILL HAD SNACK. CHECK YOUR WATER AS YOU DRINK ❑ ❑ ❑ ❑ ❑ ❑ ❑ ❑
SATURDAY	PROTEIN: COMPLEX CARB: SIMPLE CARB: ADDED FAT: SNACK*:	PROTEIN: COMPLEX CARB: SIMPLE CARB: ADDED FAT: SNACK*:	PROTEIN: COMPLEX CARB: SIMPLE CARB: ADDED FAT: SNACK*:	CHECK YOUR WATER AS YOU DRINK ❑ ❑ ❑ ❑ ❑ ❑ ❑ ❑
SUNDAY	PROTEIN: COMPLEX CARB: SIMPLE CARB: ADDED FAT: SNACK*:	PROTEIN: COMPLEX CARB: SIMPLE CARB: ADDED FAT: SNACK*:	PROTEIN: COMPLEX CARB: SIMPLE CARB: ADDED FAT: SNACK*:	CHECK YOUR WATER AS YOU DRINK ❑ ❑ ❑ ❑ ❑ ❑ ❑ ❑

*Remember to have a carbohydrate *and* a protein as a power snack.

Your name _____   Week beginning _____

	BREAKFAST	LUNCH	DINNER	COMMENTS & EXERCISE
MONDAY	PROTEIN: COMPLEX CARB: SIMPLE CARB: ADDED FAT: SNACK*:	PROTEIN: COMPLEX CARB: SIMPLE CARB: ADDED FAT: SNACK*:	PROTEIN: COMPLEX CARB: SIMPLE CARB: ADDED FAT: SNACK*:	CHECK YOUR WATER AS YOU DRINK ❑❑❑❑❑❑❑
TUESDAY	PROTEIN: COMPLEX CARB: SIMPLE CARB: ADDED FAT: SNACK*:	PROTEIN: COMPLEX CARB: SIMPLE CARB: ADDED FAT: SNACK*:	PROTEIN: COMPLEX CARB: SIMPLE CARB: ADDED FAT: SNACK*:	CHECK YOUR WATER AS YOU DRINK ❑❑❑❑❑❑❑
WEDNESDAY	PROTEIN: COMPLEX CARB: SIMPLECARB: ADDED FAT: SNACK*:	PROTEIN: COMPLEX CARB: SIMPLE CARB: ADDED FAT: SNACK*:	PROTEIN: COMPLEX CARB: SIMPLE CARB: ADDED FAT: SNACK*:	CHECK YOUR WATER AS YOU DRINK ❑❑❑❑❑❑❑
THURSDAY	PROTEIN: COMPLEX CARB: COMPLEX CARB: ADDED FAT: SNACK*:	PROTEIN: COMPLEX CARB: COMPLEX CARB: ADDED FAT: SNACK*:	PROTEIN: COMPLEX CARB: COMPLEX CARB: ADDED FAT: SNACK*:	CHECK YOUR WATER AS YOU DRINK ❑❑❑❑❑❑❑

HEALTHY EXPECTATIONS

Your name _____   Week beginning _____

	BREAKFAST	LUNCH	DINNER	COMMENTS & EXERCISE
FRIDAY	PROTEIN:	PROTEIN:	PROTEIN:	
	COMPLEX CARB:	COMPLEX CARB:	COMPLEX CARB:	
	SIMPLE CARB:	SIMPLE CARB:	SIMPLE CARB:	
	ADDED FAT:	ADDED FAT:	ADDED FAT:	
	SNACK*:	SNACK*:	SNACK*:	CHECK YOUR WATER AS YOU DRINK ❑❑❑❑❑❑❑❑
SATURDAY	PROTEIN:	PROTEIN:	PROTEIN:	
	COMPLEX CARB:	COMPLEX CARB:	COMPLEX CARB:	
	SIMPLE CARB:	SIMPLE CARB:	SIMPLE CARB:	
	ADDED FAT:	ADDED FAT:	ADDED FAT:	
	SNACK*:	SNACK*:	SNACK*:	CHECK YOUR WATER AS YOU DRINK ❑❑❑❑❑❑❑❑
SUNDAY	PROTEIN:	PROTEIN:	PROTEIN:	
	COMPLEX CARB:	COMPLEX CARB:	COMPLEX CARB:	
	SIMPLE CARB:	SIMPLE CARB:	SIMPLE CARB:	
	ADDED FAT:	ADDED FAT:	ADDED FAT:	
	SNACK*:	SNACK*:	SNACK*:	CHECK YOUR WATER AS YOU DRINK ❑❑❑❑❑❑❑❑

*Remember to have a carbohydrate *and* a protein as a power snack.

6

BUILDING BLOCK 4: EAT LEAN

WHICH IS THE LESSER OF TWO EVILS: FOOD GOING
TO WASTE OR FOOD GOING TO YOUR WAIST?

Fat is an essential nutrient needed in limited amounts for lubrication of your body, for transporting fat-soluble vitamins, for hormone production, and for fullness after eating. Vegetable oils contain essential fatty acids that are essential for your baby's brain development. This makes oils like olive oil and canola oil vital for your baby's health. Other sources of these critical fats are nuts, seeds, wheat germ, olives, and avocado.

To aid in the absorption of vitamin A, ten to fifteen milligrams of vitamin E are recommended daily during pregnancy and are found in prenatal vitamins that are recommended by your doctor. Vitamin E helps prevent the oxidation and breakdown of vitamin A and polyunsaturated fatty acids. About 60 percent of vitamin E in the diet comes directly from vegetable oil, margarine, and salad dressing. One tablespoon of olive or canola oil per day supplies at least fifteen milligrams of this vital vitamin.

The Truth About Fat

As vital as fat is as a nutrient, it's important to know that fat is also a concentrated way of getting excess calories and is an invitation to killer diseases! Pregnancy can give a sense of freedom to eat fat-laden foods with abandon. After all, you feel huge anyway! You're eating for two, right?

Remember that there is a big difference between being fat and being pregnant! The healthy foods you eat are making you and your baby healthy; the excess fat you eat only breeds more work for you after delivery. Excess fat in the diet also contributes to morning sickness and heartburn in pregnancy—that's reason enough to be cautious!

Vital Facts About Fat

- Excess fat contributes to morning sickness and heartburn in pregnancy.
- Excess fat increases your risk of cancer, particularly breast and colon cancer.
- Excess fat intake increases your cholesterol and your risk of heart disease and stroke.
- Excess fat, particularly saturated fat, elevates blood pressure.
- Excess fat increases your risk of gallbladder disease.
- Excess fat fed to animals with a genetic susceptibility to diabetes made them far more likely to develop the disease. People with a family history of diabetes should consider cutting their fat intake as one step in preventing this disease in their own lives.
- Excess fat helps make you fat! One ounce of fat supplies twice the number of calories as an ounce of carbohydrate or protein.

Rating the Fats
Dairy Foods

High Fat: (8 or more grams per serving)
CHEESE: American, blue, Brie, Camenbert, cheddar, brick, Swiss
CREAM: whipping, half-and-half, commercial sour
MILK: whole milk, whole milk yogurt
Medium Fat: (4 to 7 grams per serving)
CHEESE: farmer's, feta, mozzarella, Light Philadelphia, part-skim cheddar, part-skim ricotta, string cheese, creamed cottage cheese
MILK: 2 percent milk
Low Fat: (3 or fewer grams per serving)
CHEESE: low-fat cottage cheese, Laughing Cow nonfat cheese, nonfat ricotta
MILK: 1 percent or skim milk, nonfat plain yogurt

Meats, Fish, Poultry, and Legumes

High Fat: (8 or more grams per serving)
bacon, commercial peanut butter, corned beef, duck, frankfurters, goose,
ground meat, lunch meats, pepperoni, sausage, spareribs, tuna (packed in oil)
Medium Fat: (4 to 7 grams per serving)
beef (rib roast, steak), eggs, ham, lamb chops,
pork chops, liver, veal cutlet
Low Fat: (3 or fewer grams per serving)
chicken, clams, crab, fish, lean beef (flank, round),
legumes, oysters, scallops, shrimp, tuna (packed in water)

Sauces and Toppings

High Fat: (8 or more grams per serving)
avocado, butter, coconut, mayonnaise, margarine,
olives, oils, shortening
NUTS: almonds, pecans, cashews, walnuts
Medium Fat: (4 to 7 grams per serving)
salad dressings
NUTS: Brazil, peanuts
Low Fat: (3 or fewer grams per serving)
light sour cream, light mayonnaise, no-oil salad dressings

Soups

High Fat: (8 or more grams per serving)
all cream soups, all chunky soups, pea with ham
Medium Fat: (4 to 7 grams per serving)
beef noodle, black bean, chicken noodle, chicken vegetable
Low Fat: (3 or fewer grams per serving)
low-sodium chicken, bouillon, lentil, vegetable,
bean, gazpacho, onion

HEALTHY GOAL: AS A GENERAL RULE, THE THING THAT MAKES YOU
FAT IS FAT. BUT DO NOT CONFUSE BEING PREGNANT WITH BEING FAT.

Use the substitutes that follow to help you eliminate unnecessary
fats from your diet.

Super Substitutes

Small steps that can make a big, fat difference!

- Use skim milk, nonfat plain yogurt, skim-milk cheese, low-fat or nonfat cottage or ricotta cheese, and light cream cheese instead of higher-fat dairy products.

- Remove skin from poultry before cooking; you will cut the fat by 50 percent.

- Cream soups are the most common ingredient in any casserole and the worst nutritionally. They can easily be replaced with chicken stock, alcohol-free wine, or a combination, thickened with cornstarch or arrowroot. Add your own fresh mushrooms for a healthy cream of mushroom base that so many recipes call for. For an even richer base, combine nonfat dry milk with chicken stock and thicken with cornstarch or arrowroot.

- Cold evaporated skim milk with a touch of honey and vanilla is a super whipped topping. It does take longer to whip, but the nutritional gains are worth it. You can also use two cups evaporated skim milk with one teaspoon lemon juice; chill well; then whip. Never use nondairy whipped toppings. They are chemical non-foods, loaded with saturated fat and sugar.

- Basting with butter is another frustrating recipe direction for a healthy gourmet. Adapt, instead, by basting with tomato sauce, White Wine Worcestershire, lemon juice, or stock.

- Use only natural peanut butter. It's a great choice of protein and magnesium. Avoid the commercial-type peanut butter!—it's not much more than shortening and sugar. If you have trouble switching, begin by mixing it half-and-half with natural. Gradually increase the portion of natural.

- Try using legumes (dried beans and peas) or tofu as a main dish or a meat substitute for a high nutrition, low-fat meal.

- Use canola or olive oil for salads or cooking. They are valuable sources of monounsaturated fat, but they are still fat—so use sparingly. You can cut the amount called for in a recipe by two-thirds without sacrificing quality (i.e. three tablespoons of oil may be cut to one tablespoon), and, depending on the recipe, oils may be cut out altogether if cooking spray is used.

• Purchase tuna packed in water rather than in oil.

• Use nonstick sprays and nonstick skillets that enable you to brown meats without grease. Sauté ingredients in stocks and broths rather than fats and oils.

• Dilute soy sauce or tamari sauce half-and-half with water, and then add one teaspoon lemon juice. It increases the flavor and reduces the salt. You may also use low-sodium soy sauce.

• If using canned or frozen fruits, use only unsweetened, without sugar, packed in its own juices.

• Use more vanilla and spices in recipes. This will enable you to cut down more on the sugar since vanilla and spices enhance the impression of sweetness and flavor and have almost no calories.

• Healthy bread crumbs can be made by processing toasted whole-wheat bread in a food processor or blender.

• Use whole grains anytime a recipe calls for white. Use brown rice or whole-wheat pasta instead of white, whole-grain crackers instead of saltines.

• Substitute fiber and water for laxatives. A laxative isn't the healthy way to get rid of anything—fiber and water are!

* Use two egg whites in place of one whole egg. Egg whites are pure protein, and egg yolks are pure fat. You may want to try some of the egg substitutes on the market now.

• Eat more fish and white meats, and fewer red meats. If you eat red meats, buy them lean and trim them well of all visible fat, before and after cooking. Cook meat in such a way that diminishes fat, such as grilling or broiling on a rack.

- Rarely, if ever, eat organ meats such as liver, sweetbreads, and brains. They are loaded with cholesterol and other undesirable substances.

- Skim the fat from soup stocks, meat drippings, and sauces. Refrigerate and remove the hardened surface layer of fat before reheating.

- Order topping fats "to the side" in restaurant meals, and choose to apply them in small quantities. The typical restaurant meal contains the fat equivalent of twelve to fourteen pats of butter—in the sauces, fats, and spreads.

- Great potato toppings: salsa, nonfat sour cream, plain nonfat yogurt, blended-till-smooth nonfat cottage cheese, chives, grated Parmesan.

- Use puréed cooked vegetables, such as carrots, potatoes, or peppers to thicken soups and stews instead of creams, egg yolks, or roux.

- Use small amounts of fattier foods that pack a powerful flavor punch: feta cheese, Parmesan, coconut, toasted nuts, and turkey bacon or turkey sausage. You can cut the quantity a traditional recipe calls for in half.

7

Building Block 5: Eat Bright

Anyone can count the seeds in an apple, but only God can count the apples in a seed.

The best way to assure your vitamin intake is to go for wholegrain carbohydrates whenever possible and choose meals full of a variety of brightly colored fruits and vegetables.

Vegetables and fruits are simple carbohydrates that provide a storehouse of vitamins, minerals, and other substances for vitality living. They are also valuable sources of fiber and fluids. The fiber serves as a sort of "timed-release" capsule, releasing the carbohydrate energy into the bloodstream slowly and evenly.

Color Power

You may not be able to tell a book by its cover, but you can sure choose a healthy fruit or vegetable by its color. Generally, the more vivid in color the fruit or veggie is, the more essential nutrients it holds for you and your baby. That deep orange-red color of carrots, sweet potatoes, apricots, cantaloupe, and strawberries is a sign of their vitamin A and beta carotene content. In addition to vitamin C and iron, dark green leafy vegetables like greens, spinach, romaine lettuce, broccoli, and Brussels sprouts are also loaded with the extra bonus of being *the* source of folic acid, a "must have" in pregnancy.

Although all vitamins are needed during pregnancy in increased amounts, folic acid is the vitamin hero. It is critical for protein metabolism, particularly in periods of rapid growth. The need for folic acid nearly doubles in pregnancy to four hundred micrograms per day, so a supplement is usually recommended. In addition, you can meet your need for this valuable nutrient by having two servings of fresh, or cooked tender-crisp, dark green leafy veggies each day. Remember—if they're loaded with color, they're loaded with nutrition.

Daily choose a wide variety of fruits and vegetables, and have at least five servings each day. Depend on brightly colored fresh fruits and veggies, rather than supplements alone, to meet your baby and body's advanced needs for nutrition. Why? Despite all the laboratory wizardy, science cannot begin to uncover all the vital, baby-building substances created for us in food. The only way to give your baby their benefit is to eat the foods themselves.

High Vitamin-C Foods (have two servings each day)

1 cup blackberries or raspberries	$^2/_3$ cup cooked broccoli
1$^1/_2$ cups shredded cabbage	or $^3/_4$ cup cooked cabbage
$^1/_4$ small cantaloupe	$^3/_4$ cup cooked cauliflower
1 cup cooked collard greens	$^1/_2$ grapefruit
$^1/_2$ cup grapefruit juice	2 small oranges
$^1/_2$ cup orange juice	$^1/_2$ cup chopped papaya
$^1/_2$ red sweet pepper	3 cups raw spinach
$^1/_2$ cup strawberries	1$^1/_2$ large tomatoes
1 cup tomato juice	$^3/_4$ cup V-8 juice

Choose Variety

- Eat at least one vitamin-A rich (dark green or bright orange) selection a day. These vividly colored veggies and fruits supply you with beta carotene, which is vital for cell growth, healthy skin, bones, and eyes.
- Eat at least two vitamin-C rich (citrus, broccoli, red peppers, mango) selections with meals each day. Both you and your baby need this nutrient for tissue building and repair—for your baby's growth and strong bones and teeth.
- Eat at least two high-fiber selections (prunes, legumes) each day.
- Eat at least one cruciferous (broccoli, Brussels sprouts, cabbage, cauliflower) vegetable each day.

A Guide to Fabulous Fruits and Vibrant Vegetables

Apples: Should be firm and crisp without a watery, soft give.

> Excellent for eating: Braeburn, Red and Golden Delicious, Elstar, Fuji, Granny Smith, McIntosh, Jonathan, Winesap

> Excellent for cooking: Golden Delicious, Rome Beauty, Cortland, Granny Smith, McIntosh (never Red Delicious, as they are too dry)

> *Hint: Drizzling cut apples with lemon juice will prevent browning.*

Apricots: Should be fat and golden. Easiest to find in dried form. Very high in potassium and vitamin A.

Avocados: Use sparingly since avocados are a source of fat. They are ripe when soft to the touch and skin is darkened.

Bananas: Are considered ripe when covered with brown specks. Once ripe, refrigeration will keep them in excellent eating condition for another three to five days. (Skin may brown completely.) Bananas are very high in potassium. They are best for use as a sweetener when very brown and ripe.

> *Hint: If using in fruit salad, top the salad with sliced bananas just before serving and sprinkle with lemon juice to prevent browning.*

Berries: Sweet packages of nutritional power. Berries should be firm when purchased; avoid stained containers.

Cantaloupe: Very high in vitamins A and C, also potassium. The outside should be dull, creamy yellow when purchased, and the blossom end should be slightly soft when ripe. Look for pronounced lacy netting.

Coconut: Use sparingly since it is a source of fat. Most natural food stores have unsweetened flaked coconut. For fresher flavor, soak in small amount of milk before cooking.

Figs: Should be ripe (soft when squeezed) and plump; should smell sweet, not sour. Refrigerate.

Grapefruit and oranges: Should be round, heavy for their size and thin-skinned.

Grapes: Choose a ripe bunch. Do not ripen off the vine. The point where the grape attaches to stem should be strong and fresh, and grapes should have a full color.

Honeydew: Should have a soft blossom end; skin should be slightly sticky.

Kiwi: Should yield slightly to the touch.

Mangoes: Should yield slightly to the touch but should not be soft.

Nectarines, peaches, and pears: Are ripe when slightly soft at stem end and yellowish rather than greenish. Peaches and nectarines should have a pink blush as well.

Hint: To help with the ripening, place nectarines, peaches, pears, or plums in a brown paper bag with a banana. As the banana ripens, it releases a natural gas that ripens the other fruit as if it were still on the tree. Check daily for a fragrant smell and soft touch around the stem. When ripe, you may refrigerate.

Papaya: Should be mostly yellow, should yield slightly to pressure, and have a pleasant aroma.

Pineapple: Is ripe when it has deep green leaves at the crown, heaviness for its size, and a sweet aroma (not fermented or acidic). It should yield slightly when pressed with finger.

Plums: Should not be rock-hard, but plump and firm to the touch.

Watermelon: Should be purchased with a smooth surface, dullish sheen, and a creamy yellow underside.

Asparagus: Remove rough ends before cooking; stand in boiling water. Steam five minutes uncovered, then seven to ten minutes covered. Season with chives, garlic, lemon juice, or parsley.

Green beans: Wash and snap ends off. Steam eight to ten minutes until crisp tender. Season with basil, dill, garlic, lemon, parsley, or rosemary.

Beets: Scrub well; do not peel. Steam twenty to thirty minutes until crisp tender. Season with basil, cloves, mint, or tarragon.

Broccoli: Pare stalk of tough skin before cooking. Steam eight to twenty minutes until crisp tender. Season with garlic, lemon juice, pimento, or vinegar.

Brussels sprouts: Cut off stems and slash stem ends for quicker cooking. Steam twelve minutes. Season with chives or nutmeg.

Cabbage: Core and cut into wedges or quarters or shred. Steam twelve to fifteen minutes for wedges, five minutes for shredded. Season with basil, caraway seeds, dill, poppy seeds, or sage.

Carrots: Scrub thoroughly or pare; leave whole or slice. Steam ten minutes. Season with basil, ginger, mint, nutmeg, or parsley.

Cauliflower: Core and remove outer leaves; leave whole or cut into florets. Steam twelve to fifteen minutes. Season with basil, chives, nutmeg, rosemary, or tarragon.

Corn: Remove husks; remove silk; wash. Boil or steam for eight minutes. Season with celery seeds, chives, green pepper, or pimento.

Eggplant: Peel and slice; salt slices and let stand fifteen minutes; rinse well before use. Better to grill five to seven minutes or use in soups or casseroles. Season with basil, oregano, parsley, tarragon, or thyme.

Greens: Wash well; discard discolored leaves. Steam eight to nine minutes or until wilted. Season with basil, dill, oregano, onion, black pepper, or vinegar.

Mushrooms: Wash gently or wipe with damp cloth; trim stem ends. Sauté for five to seven minutes or use raw or cooked in other dishes. Season with basil, chives, marjoram, parsley, or thyme.

Okra: Wash and remove stem ends. Use in mixtures for soups and stews. Season with basil, bay leaf, onion, parsley, or thyme.

Onions: Remove outer, loosest layer of skin. Sauté three to four minutes or bake at 400 degrees for forty minutes. Season with dill, cloves, mint, parsley, and tarragon.

Parsnips: Scrub well or pare; leave whole or slice. Steam ten minutes. Season with dill, parsley, or sage.

Peas: Shell and wash. Steam six to seven minutes. Season with basil, dill, mint, parsley, or rosemary.

Potatoes, white and sweet: Scrub and remove any brown spots; do not peel. Bake one hour, or steam fifteen to twenty minutes. Season white potatoes with dill, chives, parsley, or rosemary. Season sweet potatoes with chives, cinnamon, or nutmeg.

Spinach: Wash thoroughly and remove stems. Serve raw in salads, or steam four to five minutes until wilted. Season with basil, chives, dill, garlic, lemon, or vinegar.

Spaghetti squash: Cut in half; remove seeds and place cut side down in small amount of water on a baking sheet. Bake at 350 degrees for forty-five minutes, until strands pull free with a fork. Season with basil, oregano, or parsley.

Summer squash: Wash; trim off ends. Steam or boil for six or eight minutes. Season with basil, oregano, or parsley.

Winter squash: Wash; cut in half and place cut side down on baking sheet, or peel and cut into small pieces to steam. Bake at 350 degrees for one hour or steam pieces for twenty to thirty minutes. Season with cinnamon, nutmeg, or orange peel.

Tips to retain nutrients in vegetables:

- Buy vegetables that are fresh if possible; when not possible, frozen is the next best choice. Avoid those frozen with butter or sauces.
- Buy locally grown foods, which are less likely to use pesticides. Get organic when possible.
- Buy in-season fruits and vegetables, which are higher in nutrients and generally grown in the United States.
- Use well-washed peelings and outer leaves of vegetables whenever possible because of the high concentration of nutrients found within them.
- Store vegetables in airtight containers in the refrigerator.
- Do not store vegetables in water. Too many vitamins are lost.
- Cook vegetables on the highest heat possible, in the least amount of water possible, and for the shortest time possible. Steaming, microwaving, and stir-frying are great choices for cooking methods.
- Cook vegetables until tender crisp—not mushy. Overcooked vegetables lose their flavor along with their vitamins.

8

Building Block 6: Eat Pure

A HUMAN BEING IS HAPPIEST AND MOST SUCCESSFUL
WHEN DEDICATED TO A CAUSE OUTSIDE HIS OWN
INDIVIDUAL, SELFISH SATISFACTION.

—*Benjamin Spock*

Should you "just say no" to that diet soda? How about that morning cup of coffee with all of its caffeine? And what should you sweeten that iced tea with? Honestly, there are no easy answers to the caffeine, artificial sweeteners, or other additives and preservative questions while pregnant . . . enough research has not been done and enough time has not passed for all the results to be in. What research has been done, as in the case of caffeine, has produced conflicting results. I consider the best posture to be "when in doubt, leave it out!" After all, it's only nine months—but nine months that will impact your baby's life, and yours—forever.

In the Book of Judges, an angel appeared to Samson's mother, saying: "You are going to conceive and have a son. Now see to it that you drink no wine or other fermented drink and that you do not eat anything unclean."* What a blessing to be made aware divinely that a baby is on the way before the moment of conception—and how incredible to be empowered to "purify your food and drink" from that very announcement. Not many of us have such an opportunity to know of our pregnancies in advance; we're often unaware until we are well into our second month. And in those weeks, it's possible that some "strong drink" or "unclean food" has been consumed. If, now that you know you're pregnant, you know that you did some things that you wish you hadn't, please be released of the fear and

*Judges 13:3-4

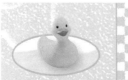

anxiety that you've harmed the baby. What is most critical is what you do *now* for the remainder of the pregnancy.

It is true that there is no safe amount of alcohol during pregnancy, but it's continuing to drink heavily throughout the pregnancy that has been associated with a wide variety of problems.

If you have been consuming large amounts of diet sodas or other caffeinated beverages, now is the time for change—it would be a healthy and wise choice to replace them with water, milk, or juices. As for the artificial sweetener question: Sugar, with all its known health problems, has been around for centuries. If you are using small amounts of sweetening—it's wise to stick with the known, rather than the unknown.

I know, I know. Easier said than done! Words are cheap—giving up unhealthy habits may seem like a high cost to pay. But you only have one chance to so dramatically impact your baby's development—why not give it your all? Even if it means giving up certain habits. If you are trying to do so without success, get some help. Speak with your health care provider, a trusted friend, your pastor, or a counselor. But do something, and do it now.

What About Alcohol?

Again, there is absolutely NO safe amount of alcohol for you to drink during pregnancy. Studies have shown that babies born to mothers who drink have lower IQs and higher rates of joint and heart defects. Even babies that are born to mothers who drink in moderation may be affected negatively—studies have shown that frequent intake of even two alcoholic drinks a day increases the risk of delivering a baby with physical and developmental problems. For some women, even smaller amounts of alcohol may produce the same risks, and "binge" drinking appears to carry an even higher risk. Research has not given us a magical quantity of what is "safe"—except none. If you choose to drink alcohol even sparingly, talk it over with your doctor.

Although alcohol use in pregnancy is the major cause of mental retardation and a leading cause of birth defects, these defects are generally preventable. The sooner a heavy drinker stops drinking during pregnancy, the less risk to her baby.

Remember: When in doubt, leave it out!

What About Caffeine?

Caffeine consumed during pregnancy has a diuretic effect, which hastens the output of body fluids and valuable calcium from the body. Caffeine triggers frequent urination. Caffeine can aggravate mood swings and interfere with restful sleep. It may also interfere with iron absorption, bad news when anemia is a none-too-distant enemy in pregnancy.

Women who have had a history of miscarriage, or who are experiencing difficulty in conceiving, are wise to cut back (or cut out) their caffeine intake. Various studies show a correlation between an increased risk of miscarriage with an increase in caffeine intake. In addition, a New Zealand study has revealed a link between high intake of caffeine (the equivalent of more than four cups of coffee per day) during pregnancy and increased risk of Sudden Infant Death Syndrome.

And be aware of this: Caffeine is a powerful addictive drug that will bring withdrawal symptoms as you give it up. Heavy users who quit "cold turkey" may experience headaches, extreme fatigue, irritability, and lethargy, which is why it's a good idea to cut back slowly over the course of a week to ten days.

Start the withdrawal process by cutting back to a more safe level of two cups of coffee or three glasses of tea. Gradually cut back, a quarter of a cup at a time, until you are down to none. Or substitute a decaffeinated product for the real thing in the same reducing amounts.

CAFFEINE IS A STIMULANT THAT ACTIVATES YOUR CENTRAL NERVOUS SYSTEM AND YOUR BABY'S. IT ACCELERATES THE BODY, CAUSING AGITATION, INCREASED HEART RATE, AND DILATION OF THE BLOOD VESSELS. A BABY DOES NOT BENEFIT FROM THIS KIND OF STIMULATION! ALTHOUGH THERE ARE NO CASES OF BIRTH DEFECTS ATTRIBUTED TO CAFFEINE INTAKE, WE DO KNOW CAFFEINE IS PASSED INTO THE BABY'S BLOODSTREAM. AN FDA STUDY ADVISES PREGNANT WOMEN TO BE PRUDENT ABOUT THEIR INTAKE. REDUCE YOUR INTAKE TO BELOW 150 MILLIGRAMS PER DAY (LESS THAN TWO CUPS OF COFFEE, TEA, OR SODA), OR, BETTER YET, GIVE IT UP ALTOGETHER.

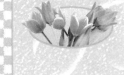

Withdrawal will be less painful if you follow the Healthy Expectations Meal Plan, eating balanced meals often. This keeps your blood sugar and energy levels up and even. In addition, try to get some outdoor exercise every day to get a boost of feel-good endorphins! And get plenty of rest.

If you decide not to cut out caffeine altogether—don't fall into fear and despair. The evidence does not show any dangers in an intake of less than two cups of caffeinated beverages a day. Just don't get java from a gourmet coffee shop—it just might give you the jitters! New analysis shows that these specialty brews can contain two to three times the caffeine found in a cup made from your typical supermarket brands.

Java and other specialty coffee drinks are stronger because more grounds are used to give the brew its rich flavor and the beans are often roasted, making the coffee even more potent. In fact, one large cup of specialty coffee packs a walloping two hundred eighty milligrams of caffeine, and some have been reported at five hundred fifty milligrams (see "How Much of a Jolt" on the next page).

Just remember: Caffeine is in lots of places—coffees, cocoa, colas, many sodas, chocolate, and many over-the-counter prescriptions. Again, the watch-phrase is: *If in doubt, leave it out!*

HOW MUCH OF A JOLT?

PRODUCT	MILLIGRAMS OF CAFFEINE
5 oz. automatic drip coffee (1 small cup)	110–150
coffee bar brews	280–550
5 oz. instant coffee	40–110
5 oz. decaffeinated coffee	2–5
5 oz. cup of tea	50–90
12 oz. glass iced tea	0–75
12 oz. can iced tea	35
decaffeinated iced tea	0
5 oz. cup hot chocolate	10
1 oz. milk chocolate	5
1 oz. baking chocolate	35
12 oz. Mountain Dew	55
12 oz. Mr. Pibb, Mellow Yellow, Surge, Sunkist Orange	42
12 oz. Coca-Cola, Tab	45
12 oz. Pepsi, Dr. Pepper, RC Cola	35
12 oz. Diet-Rite	35
12 oz. 7-Up, Sprite, Root Beer, Fresca, Ginger Ale, Diet Sunkist Orange	0
Over-the-counter medications (standard dose): No Doz, Vivarin, Caffedrine, Dristan	30
Anacin, Midol	64
Excedrin	130
Dexatrim, Dietac	200

What About Drugs?

Drugs that you take go directly to your baby's bloodstream through the placenta and can cause damage to your developing baby. Never use a drug of any kind unless your doctor has prescribed or approved it. Remember that even simple aspirin can interfere with your baby's blood supply and lengthen your labor, so check with your doctor for an okay even for what seems to be insignificant medication. When in doubt, leave it out!

What About Artificial Sweeteners?

A major controversy about the use of artificial sweeteners while pregnant comes into play as you start looking toward decreasing

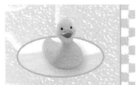

your intake of sugar. There are no absolutes in the safety of chemicals—be it saccharin, aspartame, or any new one to come. It will be years before we have all the answers.

In the case of aspartame (marketed as NutraSweet), years of study point to its safety. Yet in the short time since it has appeared on the market, cautions concerning its use have accelerated with questions about its allergic reaction in some, its danger with possible breakdown in hot foods, and its effect on children and the unborn. The battle will continue, for even though aspartame is made from natural sources, it is still made in a laboratory and is not found in nature. There are endless possibilities for problems to occur with its frequent use. As bad as sugar is, and with all of the health hazards indicated in its overuse, at least it's not chemical, and it's been used for centuries.

Also understand that as long as you continue to use sugar-laden foods or sugar substitutes, you will keep your taste buds alive for sugar. The goal is to cut back on its use so that the need is not there for everything to taste sweet. Allow your taste buds to change so that the desire for sweetness can be met in a safe way, from fruits and other naturally sweet foods that are God's natural outlets for our inborn sweet preference. *When in doubt, leave it out!*

New Days, New Ways

But old habits are hard to break—even with the knowledge that you have a precious little one within who is counting on you to be the gatekeeper—and to just say *no* to anything that could be harmful.

1. *Identify the why of change.* The only way to turn a belief into a living reality is through passion. Refuse to look at what you should or should not do—it

is impossible to be passionate for long about a list of rules. Sin-consciousness keeps peoples' eyes on the behavior they are trying to avoid rather than on the new way of living life, and we are destined to hit whatever we have our eyes on. Instead, keep your eyes on the vision: Nourishing your healthy body for a healthy baby.

2. *Identify and become educated on the new habits that will help you to realize your desires.* You are doing that by reading this book and by adopting the *Healthy Expectations* guidelines. To provide nutrients that build a healthy baby, you need to fuel the body with optimal foods at peak times. To protect, choose to avoid substances, chemicals, and activities that are detrimental to your baby. This fuels your passion to just say *no!*

Remember that your attitudes about eating are a significant contribution to your little one's health. Establishing a healthy relationship with food now, while you are pregnant, provides the framework for modeling a healthy attitude to your growing child about food. Once a child's eyes are watching your every move, your beliefs are being recorded. If you binge-eat when you are stressed, then you're putting an emotional charge on eating. The long-term result is an improper relationship with food, one of the root causes of eating disorders. Instead, pray for the wisdom to teach a healthy attitude about healthy food. Eating is enjoyable, satisfies hunger, and meets the nourishment needs of our bodies, but it wasn't meant to be the light of our lives.

3. *Identify—and avoid—resolve-breakers like fatigue, hunger, anger, or loneliness.* These can often be the music playing in the background of temptation! If your life response has been to eat when you're tired to get through, it is more difficult to choose to break for a nap than to reach for coffee and cookies. If you have spent a lifetime pushing anger down with food, it is more difficult to choose to journal your anger or discuss its cause when you are furious. Eating with a frenzy is more natural.

4. *Resist the "I've-blown-it-now" syndrome.* Even when you feel like you just blew it—no exercise, too much food, things you're trying to avoid—and you feel like Orca the whale, be assured that a lapse in healthy eating does not ruin all the health you have attained over these weeks. A lapse in your healthy lifestyle is just that—a lapse. Don't let it become a relapse, another relapse, and finally a collapse. Look at each meal and snack as an event—don't wrap it all into one bad day or one unhealthy weekend. Instead, get right back on track the very next meal or snack. Your body will stabilize quickly, you'll feel great, and your baby will be thanking you by the next day!

5. *Practice saying no.* Practice even in the bathroom or rearview mirror; you will find it becomes easier when you become accustomed to the word forming in your mouth!

6. *Get someone on the bandwagon with you—the ride is easier!*

9

BUILDING BLOCK 7: EAT, DRINK, AND BE HEALTHY!

WE CAN'T GIVE OUR CHILDREN THE FUTURE, STRIVE THOUGH WE MAY TO MAKE IT SECURE. BUT WE CAN GIVE THEM THE PRESENT.

Because water makes up 92 percent of our blood plasma, 80 percent of our muscle mass, 60 percent of our red blood cells, and 50 percent of everything else in our bodies, it is vitally important for health, especially in pregnancy! As the body fluids increase, so does your need for water. Remember, your baby is primarily water as well.

Water is as essential a nutrient as the other "fabulous five:" carbohydrates, proteins, fats, vitamins, and minerals. Without food a person can survive (albeit not well!) for weeks, even months. But without water, the human body can survive only three to five days.

We need eight to ten eight-ounce glasses of water each day—more if you are retaining fluid, and more if it is very hot.

Most of us, however, have grown up drinking just about anything but water. We list our favorite beverages as soda, coffee, tea, juice, Kool-aid—just about anything *but* water! Although we constantly hear that we should drink water, it's easier to reach for something else. We pay a price for this—we miss out on water's benefits.

The best way to drink water is to drink twelve to sixteen ounces after each meal and snack. Try to drink little or nothing with your meal (sip water if needed), because washing food down with water dilutes the digestive function and allows for fast eating. Eat slowly and dine.

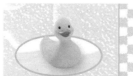

REMEMBER:
DO NOT RELY ON
YOUR THIRST MECHA-
NISM TO TELL YOU
TO DRINK WATER—
IT WILL ONLY SIGNAL
YOU TO REPLACE 35
TO 40 PERCENT OF
YOUR NEEDS. ALSO,
DON'T RELY ON YOUR
INTAKE OF OTHER
FLUIDS. NO OTHER
LIQUID WORKS LIKE
WATER. IF YOU DO
NOT TAKE IN ADE-
QUATE WATER, YOUR
BODY FLUIDS WILL
BE THROWN OUT OF
BALANCE, AND YOU
MAY EXPERIENCE
FLUID RETENTION,
CONSTIPATION,
UNEXPLAINED
WEIGHT GAIN, AND
A LOSS OF THAT
NATURAL THIRST
MECHANISM.

Water is the only liquid we consume that doesn't require the body to work to metabolize or excrete it. Even juices do not provide the solid benefits of pure, wonderful water, since they require our bodies to process the substances they contain. With soft drinks, even diet ones, our bodies have to work overtime to process and excrete the chemicals and colorings.

Water is critical for maintaining proper fluid balance. With proper protein and salt intake, water works to excrete excess stores of fluid, much like priming a pump. It is *the* natural diuretic; no other beverage works like water. It reduces excessive swelling and the risk of urinary tract infections. Water also rids your body of toxins and waste products.

Many other beverages, particularly caffeine-containing ones, actually remove more water than contained in the beverage itself. Furthermore, coffee, tea, and some sodas contain tannic acid, a product that interferes with iron and calcium absorption and competes for excretion with other bodily waste products such as uric acid. This is one reason why a glass of tea or coffee—although fluid-based—just doesn't do the job. I often call these beverages *polluted water*.

Being a mild laxative, water allows proper bowel function and waste elimination. It actually activates the fiber you eat, allowing it to pass through the gastrointestinal tract easily and quickly. Without proper water, fiber can become a difficult-to-pass glue in your colon. You may want to try a glass of warm water with the juice of a lemon; it's a mild, natural diuretic and laxative.

If you are drinking tap water, you may find its taste and safety will improve by refrigerating it for twenty-four hours or by boiling it for one minute to remove the chlorine. There has been a link found between chlorinated-water intake and a higher risk for miscarriage. You can also invest in a carbon filter for your kitchen sink. (Be sure to follow the manufacturer's directions for replacing the filters to keep them bacteria-free.) And you may find that you enjoy bottled water, club soda, or seltzer water as an alternative.

ACTION STEP 4: REVIEW YOUR EATING AND DRINKING PATTERN FOR THE LAST THREE DAYS. HOW MUCH WATER HAVE YOU BEEN DRINKING COMPARED TO HOW MUCH YOUR BODY NEEDS? CHECK A BOX ON THE SAMPLE DIARY FOR EACH EIGHT-OUNCE GLASS OF WATER THAT YOU DRINK.

Water Safety

Other than concerns about chlorine by-products, most tap water in the United States is safe and drinkable—for you and your baby. The exceptions are water sources that are contaminated with lead by passing through old lead pipes, newer pipes connected with lead soldering, or water from a well with a pump that is made with lead alloys.

To assure the safety of your water check with your local EPA or health department about the purity and safety of your community's drinking water. If you lack confidence in the answers, you can also have your water tested privately. The agencies mentioned above can give you the names of testing laboratories.

If you discover lead in your water and can identify the source, you will want to either invest in a reverse-osmosis-type filter for the household or drink bottled water. If the lead levels are low, one of the simple countertop filters or those that attach to your faucet may be adequate to get the lead out.

If you choose to go the bottled water route, be aware that just because water is bottled and packaged to look pure and safe, it isn't necessarily so. Buy spring or purified water from companies you trust. A bottle labeled "drinking water" may just come from your municipal water system—you would do just as well turning on your faucet.

HEALTHY GOAL: FOCUS ON DRINKING WONDERFUL, ESSENTIAL WATER AND DRINK ENOUGH—EIGHT TO TEN EIGHT-OUNCE GLASSES EACH DAY! DO NOT ALLOW ANYTHING TO BECOME A SUBSTITUTE FOR THE BEVERAGE YOUR BODY LIKES BEST—THE BEVERAGE OF CHAMPIONS.

10

Building Block 8:
Eat to Build

Parenting is giving your children two lasting gifts: roots and wings.

The minerals of the hour in pregnancy are calcium, iron, zinc, and sodium. Generally we eat too much sodium and not enough of the other three. While pregnant, excess sodium in the diet is to be avoided—but a major focus should be placed on getting a more than adequate intake of the minerals that build a strong body and keep you strong at the same time.

Boning Up on Calcium

Calcium is necessary to keep your own bones and teeth strong and is needed for the skeletal development in your baby. Every hour of the day throughout your pregnancy, your baby draws calcium from your body's supply. If you do not eat adequate food sources of calcium to supply the need—and 50 percent of women do not—your baby will draw from your reserves, threatening the strength of your bones. This begins the long-range risk of osteoporosis, and the short-range symptoms of inadequate calcium intake will be seen in sleeplessness, irritability, muscle cramps in the legs, uterine pain, and, possibly, higher blood pressure.

Eating enough high-calcium foods is particularly crucial in the last three months of pregnancy when the baby's bone formation is taking place at an accelerated rate. You will need at least twelve hundred milligrams of calcium each day to cover this need, and it can easily be obtained by eating four to five servings of high-calcium foods each day of your pregnancy.

WHAT ARE HIGH-CALCIUM FOODS?

PORTION EQUALING 1 SERVING OF HIGH-CALCIUM FOOD (250 MG. OF CALCIUM)

milk or nonfat yogurt . . . . .1 cup

cheese . . . .$1^1/2$ oz.

cottage cheese . . . .$1^1/2$ cups

part-skim ricotta or high-calcium cottage cheese . . . .$^1/2$ cup

salmon, canned . . . . .5 oz.

collard or turnip greens . . . . .1 cup

broccoli . . . . .2 cups

tofu or fortified soy milk . . . . .1 cup

dried beans, cooked . . . .$2^1/2$ cups

What If I'm Milk Intolerant?

Remember, it's not milk you and your baby need—it's calcium. Though milk is a convenient way to get the calcium and a great source of low-fat protein, there are many other foods that fill the bill.

There are many choices for you. The question is, "Just how intolerant are you?" Many lactose-intolerant moms will handle milk better in pregnancy, particularly in the second and third trimesters—and most can tolerate other dairy products that have had the lactose processed out, such as cheese, yogurt, or lactose-reduced milk. Many also can use most dairy products as long as they carry a capsulized form of lactase with them—a product such as "Lactaid."

If you can't tolerate any dairy products, or just plain don't like them, you can more than meet your need for calcium by choosing the nondairy foods on the list. If it's a taste bud issue, try fooling the buds with special concoctions like fresh fruit shakes with vanilla (berries and bananas are especially delicious), or try cooking your hot cereal in milk. The recipes on pages 111–119 will help to guide you in this direction. If your best efforts to include calcium-rich foods fail, be sure to get help in getting the proper amount from a calcium supplement. It's just too important to let slip.

Your prenatal vitamin/mineral will generally only contain the equivalent of one serving of a high-calcium food, so don't feel your needs are covered by this supplement. If you need to supplement further, you will do best taking additional calcium at bedtime with a small balanced snack. The two best forms for absorption are calcium carbonate and calcium citrate. Two calcium preparations, dolomite and bone meal, have been found occasionally to be contaminated with lead and should be avoided completely.

Iron-Clad Truths

Along with your needs for protein, zinc, and calcium increasing, you must be careful to eat enough foods high in iron. More than 90 percent of women may be slightly anemic before they become pregnant, and about 20 percent (one out of five) must be treated for severe iron-deficiency anemia during their pregnancy. Don't be one of these!

During the last trimester of the pregnancy, your baby will store enough iron for the first few months of life. If you do not take in enough iron each day to build your iron stores sufficiently, your baby will draw from your reserves and leave you iron-deficient and anemic. When anemic, you don't produce as many red blood cells, resulting in less oxygen circulating throughout your system. This means you may feel constantly out of breath, dizzy, weak, or you may tire easily and be more susceptible to infections. In addition, your baby will be more prone to anemia in the first year of life.

The *Healthy Expectations* eat-right prescription (small meals of high-energy, whole-grain carbohydrates and power-building, low-fat proteins complemented by brightly colored fruits and vegetables, at least every three hours) not only provides you with high-iron foods, but will also help you absorb iron most efficiently.

Because so much iron is needed during pregnancy, a supplement is almost always prescribed by your physician as a form of insurance. The most efficiently absorbed forms of iron are ferrous gluconate and ferrous fumarate and are utilized best when taken with your power snacks between meals.

Include food sources highest in iron, most notably: dried apricots, prunes, prune juice, dried beans, whole grains, well-cooked oysters and clams, and lean red meats and poultry. In addition, follow these tips for the best absorption and use:

Preventing Anemia

- Eat small frequent meals throughout the day. This allows the body to best absorb iron. The more iron you put in at one time, the less your body absorbs.
- Be sure your minimeals include a protein; it enhances your iron absorption.
- Eat fruits high in vitamin C (citrus, strawberries, and pineapple) and vegetables from the cabbage family (broccoli, cabbage, and cauliflower) at your meals and snacks; vitamin C increases your absorption of iron.
- Avoid drinking tea, colas, and coffee with your meals and snacks as these contain tannic acid, which hinders your absorption of iron. Drink refreshing, pure water instead.

FOODS HIGH IN IRON

most dried beans

clams

lean beef and veal

dark green leafy vegetables

peanuts

dried fruits (especially apricots, raisins, and prunes)

tuna, shrimp, and sardines

poultry

whole grains and cereals

Zinc Facts

Zinc is another important mineral for fetal growth and development, and you need a minimum of fifteen milligrams per day while pregnant and nineteen milligrams a day while breast-feeding. Four million Americans—most of them women of childbearing age—are deficient in zinc—daily getting only 75 percent of the RDA. This is unfortunate because, even though needed in small amounts, zinc is an essential mineral, crucial to literally hundreds of biological processes. Zinc improves muscle strength and endurance (important for labor and delivery). It provides for tissue growth and repair, as well as enhancing healing. Zinc is also involved in making genetic material, in immune reactions, and in taste and smell perceptions. (A zinc deficiency may play a part in food cravings and aversions.)

Don't feel that you have to count your milligrams to be sure you're getting your zinc each day—this amount is easily obtained through eating adequate protein evenly throughout the day. Shellfish, meat, and poultry are some of the highest food sources of zinc. Other foods rich in zinc are whole grains such as barley, beans, and nuts, and healthy vegetables such beets, carrots, and cabbage. The zinc you get from meat, fish, and poultry is more available to your body than from the other sources, particularly grains. Grains contain a substance called phytates, which may hinder zinc absorption. For this reason, vegetarians are at higher risk for zinc deficiency and should be sure to supplement properly.

In addition, if you were underweight at the beginning of your pregnancy, your physician may place particular focus on a zinc supplement for you. There is strong evidence that zinc supplementation helps to prevent underweight mothers from having premature, low-birth-weight babies.

11

BUILDING BLOCK 9:
EAT FOR ENERGY

DOING NOTHING, NOW THAT IS TIRESOME! YOU
CAN'T STOP AND REST.

Her day starts early—very early—and she wakes up tired. The alarm goes off at 4:45 A.M., and the morning routine gets started. Kids out of bed and out the door, lunches packed, and the schedule packed fuller still. "By 8:00 A.M., I'm already exhausted and feeling like I've put in a full day—then I realize that I still have a full day ahead," thirty-two-year-old Sara laments. "By 5:00 P.M., the time I want to be at my best for the people I love, I'm cranky, irritable, and craving sweets. By 8:30 in the evening, I'm on the couch in a coma. I finally stumble to bed, only to be awakened at 1:00 A.M. by the baby doing aerobics! I don't just *want* energy, I *need* energy—I don't think I can go on this way!"

Sara, a working mother of two with another one on the way, is not alone. We all need energy that lasts as long as our days last. And we desire the side benefits of energy—sharpened concentration, enduring memory, high productivity, a bright attitude, a hopeful perspective, and stress resiliency. That is the "right stuff" we need to live effective, fulfilled lives. But from where are these precious commodities going to come?

Pregnancy is a time of incredible demand on the body. For an overflow of energy, you must give yourself the supply to meet these demands and then some!

Remember the power of fueling with the eat-right prescription:

right foods at the right time and in the right balance—with lots of brightly colored fruits and veggies. And remember the secret of power snacking—food throughout the day keeps fatigue at bay! Your personal sinking spells can be prevented by eating smaller amounts of food more evenly spread throughout the day. In pregnancy, blood sugars will normally crest and fall every two-and-one-half to three hours. As they begin to fall, so will your energy, mood, concentration, and your ability to handle stress. If you've starved all day, the drop in sugar will be a "free fall," leaving you sleepy and craving sweets.

The Healthy Expectations Meal Plan (pages 82–85) will guide you into the eat-right prescription, using food as fuel to get your body working at its healthy best.

Sugar: How Sweet It Isn't!

Contrary to much popular literature, sugar is not "white death;" its darkest crime is its robbing effect on wellness. And it has partners in crime: Sugar-laden treats are loaded with saturated fats and calories as well. Generally, these treats prevent us from choosing other foods that contain nutrients like iron, chromium, and protein that work to stabilize our body chemistries. Because of the massive hormone changes in pregnancy, moms-to-be with a tendency toward fluctuating blood sugars are further affected by a roller-coaster ride of lifts and falls. The result is a wide-range effect on personality, attention span, mental performance, sleep patterns, GI function, and energy levels.

This is where Meghan, a self-professed sugar-addict-in-waiting, found herself—feeling that even the occasional eating of high-sugar foods was impossible for her because she was hurt by even "just a little bit." It wasn't about the calories or sugar's health risk; it was the effect it had on her body. The seesaw effect resulted in a the-more-she-has-the-more-she-wants syndrome that was enhanced by a programmed guilt response.

Here's how it works: When memories, moods, or availability trigger a heavy sugar intake—it brings a pleasurable rise in body chemistries that will be followed by a quick fall a few hours later. That dip triggers "eating for a lift" to relieve the fatigue, brain fog, and mood drop. Usually the food is again high in sugar, and the seesaw effect continues. Then the guilt tapes begin to play—*you've already blown it, go ahead and finish the cookies*—before you get started "back" to healthy eating again. The lapse becomes a relapse, then another relapse, and ultimately a collapse.

Your key to freedom is coming to know yourself and the power that breaks you free from any food trap. It may be necessary to "just say no" to sugar-laden foods for long enough (twelve to fourteen days) to allow your blood-sugar levels to stabilize and to allow your energy and appetite for healthy foods to return. Keep your body operative from a point of strength physically by "power snacking" every two to two-and-one-half hours throughout the day. Food throughout the day keeps your energy up and a ravenous appetite away! Keep power snacks available wherever you are—they will serve as a lift to your body and prevent the drowsiness and sweet cravings that often follow meals.

Paul told the Corinthians, "'Everything is permissible for me'— but not everything is beneficial. 'Everything is permissible for me'—but I will not be mastered by anything."* These inspired words help us to understand that while we are free to eat any food, not every food is beneficial, especially if it takes a seat of power in our daily lives.

HEALTHY GOAL: CUT BACK ON YOUR DAILY USE OF SUGAR OR SWEETS AND EAT FRUIT TO SATISFY YOUR NATURAL CRAVING FOR SUGAR. SWEET TREATS ARE NOT WORTH ROBBING YOURSELF OF YOUR PRECIOUS ENERGY AND STAMINA.

*1 Corinthians 6:12

ENERGY-ROBBER CHECKLIST

If you're too tired to even *think* about why you are—don't be too quick to blame all your exhaustion on stress. Ask yourself these questions:

Am I following the Eat Well—Live Well *prescription?* Are you eating the right foods, at the right time, in the right balance, with lots of brightly colored fruits and vegetables? Start your day with breakfast, and eat evenly distributed "minimeals" throughout your day.

Am I exercising? Instead of depleting your resources, exercise increases your energy. Just as it makes your metabolism and heart work better, exercise helps the brain function more efficiently. It also has a powerful antidepressant effect to chase the blues away by boosting endorphins.

Am I sleeping enough? Aim for eight hours of sleep each night.

Am I overdoing caffeine? Although caffeine will bring you up—for the moment—it's guaranteed to let you down hard. And, in addition to the lingering concerns about caffeine's impact on your developing baby, it also interferes with your sleeping, preventing you from getting the restful, replenishing sleep that overstressed bodies need.

Am I drinking too little? Too little *water,* that is. Many people walk around slightly dehydrated, and that can make them extremely tired—dehydration is the number one factor in fatigue. Dehydration is enhanced by climate-controlled indoor air, caffeine-overuse, and exercise. Drink at least eight to ten eight-ounce glasses of water each day.

Am I getting outside? Lack of light can make many people feel sad and tired. Taking a walk in the morning or midafternoon—even on a cloudy day—can give you some of the light you need.

Am I overdoing sweets? Excessive sugar consumption can put your energy levels on a roller coaster—giving a quick lift followed by a hard drop. Most importantly, sweet snacks often replace the very foods that can strengthen energy levels.

12

Building Block 10: Eat to Gain—the Smart Weigh

Pregnancy defined: Getting company inside one's skin.

"L et's see how that weight is doing." These were the words that Meredith dreaded almost as much as the scale experience that followed. She was in her doctor's office for her sixth-month prenatal visit, and it was right after the holidays.

Meredith had been preparing herself for this moment for two days—eating little to nothing, drinking dieter's tea. She was wearing her thinnest dress on one of the coldest days of the year, hoping to shave a few ounces off the scale's report. She went to the bathroom right before her name was called and wore slip-on sandals to quickly slip off.

"One fifty-two!" the nurse chided. "Dr. Adams is *not* going to be happy with a seven-pound weight gain in just a month. How many Christmas cookies did you eat?" As the nurse put her into the examining room, Meredith sank further into a black hole. What was she going to do about her weight? Maybe she could try one of the new herbal diet pills . . . maybe she should add an extra aerobics class . . . maybe a juice fast.

Thankfully, Meredith was open enough with Dr. Adams to ask him these very questions—and he was insightful enough to sense her desperation and see the dangers—and refer her to me for a nutrition assessment. I found that Meredith had actually gained too little weight for her stage of pregnancy, yet her efforts to control it were putting both herself and her little one at serious nutritional risk. Diet brews, starvation, and such spell danger to anyone, especially a pregnant someone.

I've worked with hundreds of Merediths—women who have always kept their weight tightly gripped in their control, but who were now pregnant. It seems that one of the first questions I'm asked by any newly pregnant person is about weight gain. To many it seems to be the "bottom line" in nutrition during pregnancy—and a subject that brings great confusion and fear.

My answer to the weight-gain question is a simple one: The healthiest babies are born to women who allow themselves a natural weight gain during pregnancy. No matter what your weight was before you conceived, you must have additional nutrient intake to support an increase in your own body's metabolism, plus the growth of your baby.

You may have been directed differently with past pregnancies, or you may hear conflicting reports from your mom or aunts. It is very important to remember that each generation has its own set of rules for pregnancy, and your mother's rules (even though "you and your sister turned out just fine!") are not your rules. Remember, there was a time when pregnant women were encouraged to have a cocktail to relax. There was a time when women were put on dangerous diuretics to reduce swelling, and smoking was considered necessary to keep the weight gain down ("better a smoke than food"). Well, thank goodness, we've truly come a long way, baby!

When it comes to proper weight gain, this controversy has been swinging back and forth like a pendulum for years. Again, our mother's generation was held victim to the belief that the less weight gained during pregnancy the better. This misconception, widely held a few decades ago, was based on the belief that women who gained little or no weight would be less likely to develop complications during pregnancy and would have smaller, more easily delivered babies. The opposite camp, emerging in the eighties, urged women to eat to their heart's content and gain any amount of weight. Research has proven both theories wrong, and we now know that a healthy weight increase is twenty-five to thirty pounds—gained evenly throughout the pregnancy. This is the 1990 recommendation from the U.S. National Institute of Medicine.

If you were underweight before pregnancy (by less than 10 percent of your ideal weight), it's suggested that you gain a little more weight (twenty-eight to thirty-five pounds). If you are overweight (by more than 10 percent over your ideal weight) when you become pregnant, it is recommended that you gain a little less (twenty to twenty-five pounds). Less weight can be gained if there are adequate energy reserves in place before pregnancy—but the minimum weight gain is still twenty pounds. Babies whose mothers gain under twenty pounds are more likely to be premature, small for their gestational age, and to suffer growth retardation in the uterus. And although there's a good chance that a woman with an enormous weight gain may have an oversized baby, the mother's weight gain and the weight of her infant don't always correlate. It's quite common for a mother to gain sixty pounds, yet deliver a six-pound baby, and for another to gain twenty pounds, yet deliver a hefty eight-and-one-half pounder. The quality of the food that is resulting in the weight gain is more important for the health and size of the baby than just the quantity alone.

In addition, the pattern of weight gain is at least as important as the total amount. The goal is a slow steady gain—four to five pounds the first three months and approximately three to four pounds during each of the remaining six months. It's not unusual to gain a bit more in the fifth month when the baby kicks into high-growth gear, nor for the weight gain to drop off in the last two weeks. These are simple recommendations, but they are not always easy!

It is normal for your weight to fluctuate a little—gaining half a pound one week, and one-and-one-half the next. Your weight will also fluctuate throughout the day. For this reason, weigh yourself at the same time of day under the same conditions, and weigh yourself weekly, not daily! This prevents you from seeing a weight on the scale that is more related to that pint of water

THE GOOD NEWS IS THIS: IF YOU ARE EATING THE RIGHT FOODS, AT THE RIGHT TIMES, IN THE RIGHT BALANCE—EVEN WITH A FEW SPLURGES—YOU WILL NATURALLY GAIN THE RIGHT AMOUNT OF WEIGHT IN YOUR PREGNANCY. IT'S HOW YOUR BODY WAS CREATED! STAY TUNED INTO THE HEALTHY EXPECTATIONS MEAL PLAN, AND YOUR BODY—AND BABY'S—WILL THRIVE WITH THE EAT-RIGHT PRESCRIPTION.

IF PEOPLE ASK YOU HOW MUCH WEIGHT YOU'VE GAINED, SMILE AND SAY, "ENOUGH."

you just drank or seeing the weight of that heavy bathrobe. Also, only keep track of your weight on one scale. It really doesn't matter what you weigh at the grocery store; it's what you weighed last week at home compared to this week, on that same home scale. Or what you weighed last week at the doctor's office at the same time of day that you are weighing this week—without shoes.

Your overall goal is to gain as steadily as possible, without any sudden drops or gains. Be sure to check with your doctor if you don't gain, or even lose, weight for two weeks straight between the fourth to eighth month, or if you gain more than three pounds in one week during this same period—especially if it doesn't appear to be related to a change in eating patterns. If all appears to be well—and you just seem to be gaining too much—you may want to keep track of your eating for several days and compare it to the Healthy Expectations Meal Plan for modification.

Of course, the whole weight-gain picture changes for woman with special needs. I develop meal plans for my clients who begin pregnancy extremely underweight to allow them to gain enough weight during their first trimester to get them close to their ideal weight—then have them gain the needed twenty-five pounds over the remaining course of the pregnancy.

Kim was in dance on Broadway and very thin when she became pregnant. We developed a meal plan for her to gain a healthy fifteen pounds in her first trimester, and we had to work as hard on her self-image as we did her eating plan! She had to slowly let go of the dancer's body and embrace that she was growing a baby. She gained an additional twenty-three pounds throughout the second and third trimesters (a total of thirty-eight pounds) and was back to a great weight within four months. She was back to her prepregnancy weight—and dancing—after a long run of nursing!

I have also, in close teamwork with the doctors, developed careful meal plans for extremely overweight pregnant moms to allow a weight gain of only fifteen pounds. Again, this has to be done very carefully, with the highest quality of food.

Women who are carrying more than one baby need to gain significantly more weight—forty to forty-five pounds for twins, even more for more! (See page 184, "What About Multiple Births?")

Tallying the Smart Weigh

The amount of weight you gain appears to have a positive effect on your baby's health far beyond the birth weight—maybe for the baby's entire life. A healthy weight gain is not just fat weight, but is instead specific body changes that add up to weight on the scale. A twenty-eight-pound weight gain at delivery would consist of:

Your baby (average newborn weight)	7^1/$_2$ lbs.
Increased size of breasts	2 lbs.
Increased size of uterus and uterine muscles	2 lbs.
Placenta	1^1/$_2$ lbs.
Amniotic fluid	2 lbs.
Extra blood volume and maternal fluids	8 lbs.
Energy reserves	<u>5 lbs.</u>
TOTAL	28 lbs.

As you can see, the weight adds up; never confuse being pregnant with being fat. Fight notions to starve yourself in an attempt to reach an "ideal" weight, even if you are ahead of schedule in weight gain. Remember, your baby is going to gain most of his weight during the third trimester.

Never try to lose weight, or even to maintain your weight, during pregnancy! Even though you may feel that you have more than enough fat stores to feed the baby, fat stores may provide energy for you but not nutrients for your baby. Severe caloric restrictions will shortchange the baby, and you will pay the cost with your own health and impeded recovery. Restricting calories limits the chances of getting the right amount of nutrients (such as calcium, iron, and protein). When caloric intake is too low, protein will be used for energy rather than building your baby.

This can actually backfire—the protein deficit can cause your body to begin to hold fluids excessively—and the scale can sky-rocket in a very unhealthy way. This is why sudden, extreme weight gain during pregnancy should be reported immediately to your doctor. If you diet during pregnancy, your own body fat will be used for energy and will form ketones, a waste product. Ketones can be absorbed into your baby's bloodstream and may damage your baby's brain cells.

If you do find that your weight gain has gotten significantly out of the desired range, take action to get back on track. Just don't try to stop it in its tracks! Your baby can't thrive on what you've already gained but requires the weight you still have to gain.

This is your first chance to impact your baby's health directly. You will have a lifetime to lose weight! Use this time as a chance to break the "diet mentality." Learn what positive eating is all about so that it will be possible to stay in great shape and easily get back into shape after that precious baby is born. It's a side effect of eating well! What a wonderful time it is now to start leaving out sugar-laden foods and salty, high-fat snacks and start replacing them with delicious but healthy foods.

By the way, my friend Jenny always adds seven to eight pounds to her answer regarding her pre-pregnancy weight—so that it will never be recorded *anywhere* how much she really gained during the time she thought she might be pregnant and her first doctor's appointment!

Eating Disorders and Pregnancy: A Time to Heal

Kelly started her pregnancy weighing one hundred twenty pounds. That would sound good and healthy, until you know that she was a large-framed, five-foot eleven-inches—and her ideal weight was one hundred sixty-five pounds. To stay at that sleek one hundred twenty pounds she was throwing up five times a day and had done so since ninth grade.

It was Kelly's first pregnancy, and when she started to gain weight, even the first two to three pounds, she panicked—and came to see me.

Becoming pregnant raises new fears for women who have, or once had, eating disorders such as anorexia, bulimia, chronic dieting syndrome, or who are chronically using purging methods such as diuretics, laxatives, or excessive exercise. If the eating disorder continues through pregnancy, or if it is moved to action by the fear of "getting fat," serious health problems can occur—both for the mom-to-be and her unborn child. A woman who is underweight and fails to gain enough weight during pregnancy risks premature delivery and having a baby with a low birth weight as well—making it difficult for this newborn to grow and thrive.

Because more than 75 percent of those suffering with an eating disorder are women in their reproductive years, a large number obviously become pregnant—often while still in the throes of a gripping disease. For any woman, gaining weight can be distressing. Someone who has never struggled with a profound eating disorder can accept weight gain as the right thing to do and shrug it off. But for the woman with an eating disorder it can become a crisis.

Yet, this can be a magnificent time to break out of the pattern of thought and body image associated with eating disorders. Keeping the focus that this is one time to focus on the baby growing within rather than her own body and that she is providing that baby with nourishment to grow physically into a healthy, thriving child is the key for someone struggling with an eating disorder. But she's also being transformed into a mom with a healthy image about her weight and her relationship with food. For a child to be raised with good feelings about her body, it must start with Mom.

Kelly found that pregnancy enabled her to stabilize her behavior and her frenzied thinking for the first time since her teen years. It was a time of calm for her. There is some research that suggests this calm may be hormonal in nature. For Kelly, it was more. Because her eating disorder was rooted in performance and image—trying to be perfect in every way—she could revel in the truth that she was "performing" perfectly by nourishing her baby with food and love, that gaining weight was succeeding—and it was very much within her control.

It was also the first time that Kelly had really acknowledged that she had a problem with an eating disorder and sought help. This became vitally important after her baby was born and the symptoms began to return. Once again, controlling her food and purging became the tempting way to deal with the new chaos and stress of being a new mother, and a not-too-confident-one at that.

If you are struggling with this whole issue of eating and your weight, please know that it is hard to heal on your own. An eating disorder is a disease that can be treated and healed, but not just a weakness you can walk out of on your own. Share your struggle with your doctor and get a recommendation for a counselor and a nutritionist like myself.

Getting well is possible, and its rewards carry through the rest of your life, and your baby's.

Part 2

PREPARING A HEALTHY BODY
FOR A HEALTHY BABY

13

Preparing Your Body for Pregnancy

BABIES ARE SUCH A NICE WAY TO START PEOPLE.

If you are not presently pregnant, but thinking about becoming so—you are already giving the best gift you can to you and your little one. You are learning now how to prepare a healthy body for a healthy baby.

You can choose today to change the lifestyle habits—smoking, drinking, caffeine, artificial sweeteners, and drugs—that can affect your soon-to-be developing little one. This is a time to get pure and clean. Almost everything you swallow, inhale, or inject can affect your baby. Make habit changes now, before you conceive and before your body begins to undergo so many of its own physical changes. You—and your sweet precious—will reap bountifully from the changes you make today.

Because much of your baby's critical development takes place during the first few weeks after conception, prepregnancy is the time to make the difference. Most of the baby's brain-cell division occurs when a woman doesn't even know she's pregnant. Now is the time to establish a well-balanced diet, to build up nutrient stores, to start exercising regularly, and to lose or gain weight, if needed.

If you have chronic medical conditions such as allergies, high blood pressure, diabetes, or kidney disease, getting your body processes in control before you become pregnant is vital to having the healthiest pregnancy and baby possible! Get your immunizations up to date now, before you become pregnant. Ask your doctor

72

about flu shots if flu season is approaching.

Genetic counseling may be well-advised prior to pregnancy if you know that you may have an inherited disorder or birth defect— or if you are concerned that you might. Moms- or dads-to-be who have been exposed to radiation, medications, toxic chemicals, serious infections, or street drug use will benefit from genetic counseling as well. A board-certified counselor will gather assessment information including your family history and a blood sample used for chromosome studies. If problems are identified, the counselor not only provides emotional support and guidance, but he or she also can refer couples to medical specialists to meet their need.

This is even a good time to get into the habit of having someone else change the kitty litter. Toxoplasmosis is an infection that can damage your baby-to-be's central nervous system, and one of the ways it's transmitted is through exposure to cats' feces. You don't have to get rid of kitty—just beg off the clean-up!

If you are underweight, you should try to eat nutritiously to gain up to a healthy weight; women who weigh too little when they conceive are more likely to have smaller babies. Being underweight can also interfere with conception, so ask your doctor or a recommended registered dietitian to help you identify your ideal weight. Also ask for help in developing a nutritious meal plan to gain weight the smart weigh! You don't need to "fatten" up, but instead to "build up."

If you are overweight, the time to lose the extra pounds is before pregnancy, not during. If you need to lose weight, it must be done in the healthiest way possible. A fad diet or starvation is no way to prepare your body for the big event; it only leaves your body deficient of nutrients and vitamins. Good eating can cause you to lose weight as a side effect of proper nourishment, and it can energize you to get started into a routine of moderate exercise.

The Healthy Expectations Meal Plan is perfectly balanced to meet your needs and prepare your body for pregnancy. You will need to adjust portion sizes according to your weight goals. The same timing and balance of eating applies, just eating smaller portions if trying to lose weight, and more if trying to gain weight, the healthy weigh! In addition, you should begin to take prenatal vitamins containing four hundred micrograms of folic acid now. If you have been on birth control pills, you need to supplement with eight hundred micrograms of folic acid until you become pregnant.

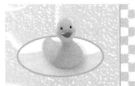

MEAL-PLANNING
STRATEGIES TO IMPROVE
FERTILITY:

• Achieve a close-to-ideal body weight.

• Avoid caffeine, due to its link to miscarriage.

• Add adequate calories, animal protein, and a prenatal vitamin/mineral supplement to a vegetarian diet.

• Get help for any hidden or overt eating disorders.

• Ensure adequate iron stores.

• Both partners should supplement diet with vitamin C, zinc, and selenium.

• Avoid alcohol.

• Drink purified or natural spring-bottled water due to tap water's link to miscarriage.

• Limit intake of barley, oats, soybeans, carrots, fennel, and green beans—all contain natural inhibitors to fertility.

• Avoid extremes in exercise.

If you have had a miscarriage in the past or have delivered a baby with birth defects—now is the time to find out how to improve the outcome of your next pregnancy and health of your next baby.

Difficulties in Conceiving

This is the day when many women are trying desperately to become pregnant. With the availability of modern tests and procedures, don't overlook the simple truth of preparing the body nutritionally. Eating well before pregnancy is much like building a home with a strong foundation, one that can firmly stand and house a very special guest.

Infertility, defined as "not conceiving after one year of unprotected intercourse," affects more than five million couples. Although some of these numbers may be a result of delaying pregnancy (generally, the older we are, the longer we need to conceive), there are any number of factors involved. Seeking assistance for infertility can be a painful, heartbreaking experience of loss.

I am often consulted in the process of couples seeking to conceive. Nutrition can, and does, play a vital role in fertility. Being underweight, with a low body fat percentage, is considered a primary cause of being unable to conceive. According to one estimate, up to 12 percent of infertility that is associated with ovulatory dysfunction is a result of being excessively underweight or overweight. This is due to the role of body fat in synchronizing hormones in such a rhythm to provide for conception. Yet, too much body fat can also be a problem; excess body fat, particularly when deposited in the breasts and abdomen, can adversely impact fertility by affecting the amount and types of circulating hormones.

I work with my patients to develop a plan to stabilize the body's chemistries and bring the weight into an ideal range through healthy eating and exercise. The plan is very focused on getting the optimum in nutritive values and the avoidance of substances that can be toxic to fertility. See the meal-planning strategies on the previous page to improve fertility for the high points of this plan. Small things can become big—certain foods (like barley, oats, soybeans, carrots, fennel, and green beans) contain natural chemicals that can inhibit fertility. Since these are often the mainstays of a strict vegetarian diet, I sometimes advise a redirection of food choices when a vegan is struggling to conceive.

I also work to develop personal strategies for the best processing of stress from the struggle to conceive and from other life situations. And yes, there has been great success—again, particularly when the inability to conceive is related to ovulatory dysfunction. Overall, embracing a plan of self-care helps in so many ways—physically, emotionally, and spiritually.

IF YOU ARE TRYING TO GET PREGNANT NOW, TREAT YOUR BODY AS IF YOU ALREADY ARE.

14

How Does Your Baby Grow: The Nine-Month Countdown

How does your baby grow?

The First Day: Today a single-cell organism was formed from the union of your ovum, or egg, and your baby's daddy's sperm. Over the coming months, your daughter or son will develop from this barely visible single cell, called a *zygote*. This beginning is called *conception*.

As you think back, do you remember this date? Some women can feel when they ovulate, while others can't. Although hundreds of sperm may swarm the egg, only one will penetrate the egg's outer surface. While this process involves a tremendous amount of activity by the involved cells, you are generally unaware of it. The incredible thing to realize is that your baby is a WINNER—beating out all the other sperm to fertilize your egg—this baby MADE IT!

The First Month: Conception usually occurs about two weeks after the beginning of the last menstrual cycle. After ovulation, the egg passes from an ovary into the fallopian tube, which is five inches long. This is where the egg is joined by the sperm. It then travels to the uterus where it implants in the uterine wall, which usually takes nine to ten days. Your precious baby is beginning to grow rapidly, doubling in size every twenty-four hours.

Only twenty days after conception, the foundation for the child's brain, spinal cord, and entire nervous system will have been established as well as rudiments of the eyes. The S-shaped, primitive heart is beginning to beat. Your baby-to-be is now one-twelfth inch long and one-sixth inch wide.

The Seventh Week: The chest and abdomen are completely formed. The mouth opens; there are tiny shell-like external ears. All of the backbone is laid down, and the spinal canal is closed over. Arms and legs are beginning to be visible. The baby is now one-half inch long and weighs one-thousandth of an ounce. What you are eating is so important to your health and your baby's development!

The Eighth Week: The embryo is now a fetus to your doctor. It is "mama's precious" to you. Color begins to appear in the eyes; jaws are now formed, and so are the teeth. Fingers and toes are present. The baby is a little over an inch long and weighs one-third ounce— smaller than an aspirin tablet.

The Twelfth Week: Your precious bundle of joy is now three inches long and weighs one whole ounce. Arms, legs, hands, feet, fingers, and toes are fully formed. Nails appear. The brain, spinal cord, and muscles connect, and the baby can kick those tiny legs even though the movement cannot be felt yet. That sweet thing can make a fist, open its mouth, and squint those eyes.

The Fourth Month: The precious baby you are nurturing is now eight inches long and weighs six ounces. The heartbeat is strong and audible with a stethoscope. The baby may occupy the time now by sucking its thumb. The skin is forming into several layers and is pink and wrinkled. The skeletal system is thickening and developing, and some digestion even begins this month. The uterus is greatly enlarging.

The Fifth Month: Your angel is ten to twelve inches long and weighs fourteen to sixteen ounces. We finally got up to a pound. Your baby is active now, and you may begin to feel the movement, known as "quickening," at about twenty weeks. A covering like peach fuzz appears over the entire body, and hair begins to grow. Internal organs are developing at an astonishing speed.

The Sixth Month: Your baby now has fingerprints and footprints as the ridges on palms and soles of feet are fully formed. It has now grown to a length of fourteen inches and weighs two pounds, which means you will gain slightly more weight than previously. You will be able to feel definite little friendly kicks as the baby makes you aware of its presence! A coating called "vernix caseosa" has formed to protect the skin from constant contact with the amniotic fluid. This vernix remains on the skin and serves as a lubricant during delivery as the baby passes through the birth canal. The eyes are open now, and the baby can hear sounds.

The Seventh Month: The weight of your child has doubled since last month. Skin is red and wrinkled, but the fatty tissue begins to form underneath it and will fill it out to make it "soft as a baby's bottom." The baby is gaining about one-half pound a week now, and by the end of this month will weigh two-and-one-half to three-and-one-half pounds and will be about sixteen inches long. The organ that develops in these last months is the brain. Brain size increases tremendously and develops into a mature brain. Your nutrition during these last months greatly affects birth weight and brain size. If born now, the baby could probably survive with special neonatal care, as the organ systems are well-developed. The next two months, however, are periods of growth to ensure adequate size for a healthy full-term delivery. It is also laying up stores of iron, so be very careful that you avoid "empty calorie" foods.

The Eighth Month: As more fat is deposited under the skin, the baby reaches about five pounds in weight and eighteen inches in length. Lungs develop strength. Soon you will hear that wailing you've been waiting for. The brain continues its rapid development, with the cells multiplying at a rapid rate. This continues to be a period of vital nutrient supply for the baby.

The Ninth Month: By delivery time your baby will weigh an average of seven pounds and measure twenty to twenty-one inches long. Your baby's biggest weight gain will occur during this last month. It will store iron, fat-soluble vitamins, and minerals as reserves after birth; it is also building up immunities. That little darling is now ready and waiting to join its family.

15

Healthy Expectations Meal Plans—While You Wait

EVERYTHING COMES TO SHE WHO WAITS, AS LONG AS
SHE WORKS WHILE SHE WAITS.

During pregnancy, especially during the first three months, your hormones are fluctuating wildly, and so is your blood sugar level. This can lead to fatigue, queasiness, and nausea. Actually, a touch of queasiness may be your first clue that you are pregnant.

The exact cause of morning sickness is simply unknown. It may be hormones affecting blood sugars and increasing gastric acids; it may be pregnancy enzymes; or it may be an increased sense of smell. It may be the emotional roller coaster and physical stress response to the reality of pregnancy. What is known is that it is not restricted to the morning. It is also known that fatigue, stress, and a diet low in vitamins, minerals, and carbohydrates can make early-pregnancy nausea even more severe. Also known, but not commonly so: An even, frequent intake of low-fat proteins balanced with carbohydrates throughout the day will help to keep your blood sugars stable and prevent the quease before it hits! Don't accept that you have to suffer the consequences of being among the unlikely numbers who are susceptible—take charge and feel good now.

Quitting the "Big Quease"

As you might have noticed, once you begin to feel bad, it's too late.

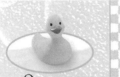

OVERCOMING MORNING SICKNESS

- Eat when you are feeling your best.

- Eat crackers before you move out of bed, and then relax for ten to fifteen minutes. Resist even getting up to use the restroom!

- Have a small glass of cool, gentle juice. Follow with breakfast.

- Eat balanced snacks and small meals of carbohydrates and protein every one-and-one-half to two hours.

- Drink water after meals and after snacks—not on an empty stomach.

- Choose foods that sound good to you, balanced wisely.

- Stay clear of strong smells.

- Keep eating often, even after you feel better.

You can prevent the blood sugar dips. Eat when you are feeling your best. Pregnant women simply feel better if their stomachs are neither too full nor too empty.

Start before you even get out of bed, when your blood sugar is the lowest, with some crackers kept at your bedside. If whole wheat is not appealing at this time, try a milder rice cracker. Relax in bed while eating them, and continue to lie still for ten to fifteen minutes. Don't get up! Follow this with some cool, gentle juice (like white grape or apple-cranberry) upon arising and a small balanced breakfast. Continue to eat small snacks and meals every one-and-one-half to two hours throughout the day and evening, including a night snack. Your night snack is the beginning of a well morning. You will also sleep more restfully and wake more refreshed.

Avoid fats in your food as much as possible, since these stay in your stomach longer and are harder to digest.

Avoid drinking liquids with meals; instead, drink after the meal, and drink a lot. Fluids are vital for keeping your body well-hydrated and working at its healthiest best—and water is the very best choice. Just avoid putting liquids, even water, on an empty stomach.

Choose foods that sound good to you—just avoid greasy, fat-laden, or fried foods that trigger more acid secretion into the stomach. Put "maybe-I-could-stomach-this" foods into a proper balance of carbohydrate and protein, no matter how bizarre the combinations may be. Go for the healthiest and lowest-fat version possible. If chips sound good, go for Baked Lays and add a piece of string cheese or lean, sliced ham for protein. Cold foods may be more appealing than hot foods, possibly due to the different "mouth-feel" and smells. A dinnertime sandwich may be tolerated much better than the classic hot fixings! Watermelon is a tolerated favorite for many—I have one mom of twins who could count on watermelon and low-fat cottage cheese with blueberries when all else failed.

Stay clear of strong smells. The enhanced sense of smell in pregnancy may have been part of God's master design to keep you out of toxic environments—and the impact of nausea is amazing. Perfumes, body odors, cooking smells, mold, mildew, diesel smells, coffee, cigarette smoke—you name it; all can be a trigger for the queasies. Become aware of your triggers, maybe by keeping a diary, and make others aware of them, too. You can't control every smell that comes your way, but you can get yourself away from it at times. You may find that this is a good time to get takeout from your favorite restaurant instead of eating in where you are trapped with the scents around you.

Speaking of smells . . . an apple a day may keep the queasies away! There's evidence that the scent of green apples can stabilize the body and prevent nausea. The sweet-tart taste of a Granny Smith may be refreshing as well! Lemons also seem to help, either by masking other smells or stimulating a chemical release in the brain. Smells do have an impact on how we feel, so go for the good ones!

Exercise works miracles for many—although it seems a stretch when you feel like you need to carry a motion-sickness bag with you on your walk! But the truth is, the resulting boost in endorphins that you receive through moderate exercise may be the lift you need.

Sea-Bands, one-inch wrist bands available at marine shops and pharmacies, have no unhealthy side effects and are often found to relieve nausea. If it works for seasickness, it just may work wonders for your morning sickness. Ginger capsules and ginger tea are also being studied to see if their anti-motion-sickness benefit impacts morning sickness as well.

Brushing your teeth frequently with a minty toothpaste or rinsing with a minty mouthwash can help to overcome the unpleasant excess saliva production that often accompanies morning sickness.

Don't take anything for your nausea—over-the-counter or from a health food store—unless it is approved by your physician. Some are unsafe, most are untested, and some may aggravate rather than help. Even your prenatal vitamin supplement may be a culprit; you may have to take it at night or stop it altogether for a short period.

Once you begin on the road to overcoming the queasies, it will take your body two to three days to stabilize. And once you begin to feel better, continue to eat small meals for peak energy and wellness. You may feel like you stay just "on the edge" of queasiness—and you may find this lasts for a number of months (the average duration of morning sickness is seventeen-and-one-half weeks). During this period of time, keep focused on right eating at the right time, setting the stage for the rest of the pregnancy.

HEALTHY GOAL: EAT SMALL MEALS EVERY ONE-AND-ONE-HALF TO TWO HOURS TO PREVENT SICKNESS, RATHER THAN EATING TO TRY TO CURE IT AFTER IT HITS. IN THE CASE OF MORNING SICKNESS, "AN OUNCE OF PREVENTION REALLY IS WORTH A POUND OF CURE!"

Just don't fall into the trap of waiting until you are weak and hungry to eat—it won't be pretty!

Follow this "No Nausea" meal plan designed to prevent morning sickness. It will take two to three days for your body to stabilize, so don't give up.

Meal Plan to Combat Morning Sickness

Before getting out of bed

5 whole-grain crackers. Relax for 10 to 15 minutes.

Upon arising

6 oz. unsweetened juice (no citrus)

Breakfast (within 1/2 hour of rising)—7:00 A.M.

COMPLEX CARBOHYDRATE: 1 slice of 100 percent whole-wheat bread OR 1/2 whole-wheat English muffin OR 1 cup cereal WITH added bran
PROTEIN: 1 oz. low-fat cheese OR 1 egg OR 6 oz. skim milk or yogurt for cereal
SIMPLE CARBOHYDRATE: 1 piece of fresh fruit

First morning snack—8:30 to 9:00 A.M.

CARBOHYDRATE: 5 whole-grain crackers OR 1 piece fruit OR 2 rice cakes
PROTEIN: 1 oz. cheese/lean meat

Second morning snack—10:30 to 11:00 A.M.

Repeat earlier snacks or / cup Trail Mix (page 19)

Lunch—12:30 to 1:00 P.M.

COMPLEX CARBOHYDRATE: 2 slices of bread OR 1 baked potato OR 10 crackers OR 1 whole-wheat pita
PROTEIN: 2 oz. cooked poultry, fish, roast beef OR low-fat cheese
SIMPLE CARBOHYDRATE: 1 small piece of fresh fruit OR 1 cup non-creamed soup
HEALTHY MUNCHIE: Raw vegetable salad, if desired
ADDED FAT: 1 tsp. mayonnaise OR 1 Tbsp. dressing

First afternoon snack—2:30 to 3:00 P.M.

Repeat earlier snack choices OR $1/2$ cup plain yogurt mixed with $1/2$ cup fruit OR 1 Tbsp. all-fruit jam

Second afternoon snack—4:30 to 5:00 P.M.

Repeat earlier snack choices

Dinner—6:30 to 7:00 P.M.

COMPLEX CARBOHYDRATE: 1 cup rice or pasta OR 1 cup starchy vegetable
PROTEIN: 2-3 oz. cooked chicken, turkey, fish, seafood, lean roast beef OR $1/2$ cup cooked beans
SIMPLE CARBOHYDRATE: 1 cup nonstarchy vegetable OR 1 piece of fruit
HEALTHY MUNCHIE: Raw vegetable salad, if desired
ADDED FAT: May use 1 tsp. of margarine/butter or olive oil, OR 2 Tbsp. sour cream OR 1 Tbsp. salad dressing

Night snack

Any power snack (page 19) or $3/4$ cup cereal with $1/2$ cup skim milk or yogurt

The Second and Third Trimester
Healthy Expectations Meal Plan

Upon arising

6 oz. unsweetened juice (such as grape, apple, cranberry)

Breakfast (within $^1/_2$ hour of rising)

COMPLEX CARBOHYDRATE: 2 slices whole-wheat bread OR 1 whole-wheat English muffin OR $1^1/_2$ cups cereal with raw bran added (begin with 1 teaspoon bran, gradually increasing to 2 tablespoons) OR 2 homemade muffins

PROTEIN: 2 ounces part-skim cheese OR 2 tablespoons natural peanut butter (limit to one time per day) OR $1^1/_2$ cups skim milk for cereal OR 2 eggs (limit whole eggs to 2 times per week) or $^1/_2$ cup egg substitute OR $^1/_2$ cup low-fat, high-calcium cottage cheese or skim ricotta OR $1^1/_2$ cups yogurt

SIMPLE CARBOHYDRATE: 1 piece fresh fruit

Morning snack

CARBOHYDRATE: 5 whole-grain crackers OR 2 rice cakes or Wasa breads AND 1 piece fresh fruit

PROTEIN: 2 ounces part-skim cheese or lean meat OR 2 tablespoons natural peanut butter (limit peanut butter to once a day) OR 1 cup nonfat plain yogurt mixed with 1 teaspoon all-fruit spread OR $^1/_2$ cup low-fat, high-calcium cottage cheese or skim ricotta

Lunch (begin with 1 piece of fresh fruit or 6 oz. juice)

COMPLEX CARBOHYDRATE: 2 slices whole-wheat bread OR 1 baked potato OR 1 whole-wheat pita bread

PROTEIN: 4 ounces part-skim cheese OR 4 ounces cooked poultry, fish, or lean roast beef OR 1 cup cooked legumes

SIMPLE CARBOHYDRATE: 1 additional serving of fresh fruit OR 1 cup noncreamed soup OR 1 cup nonstarchy vegetables

HEALTHY MUNCHIE (OPTIONAL): raw vegetable salad with no-oil salad dressing OR 1 additional serving fresh fruit OR 1 cup nonstarchy vegetables or noncreamed soup

ADDED FAT (OPTIONAL): 1 teaspoon mayonnaise (or 1 tablespoon light mayonnaise) OR 1 teaspoon butter or margarine OR 1 teaspoon olive oil or canola oil OR 1 tablespoon salad dressing

Afternoon snack

Repeat earlier snack choices OR $^1/_2$ cup Trail Mix (pg. 19)

Dinner

COMPLEX CARBOHYDRATE: $1^1/_2$ cups rice or pasta OR $1^1/_2$ cups starchy vegetable

PROTEIN: 4 ounces cooked chicken, turkey, fish, seafood, or lean roast beef OR 1 cup cooked legumes

SIMPLE CARBOHYDRATE: 1 cup nonstarchy vegetable AND 1 piece fresh fruit

HEALTHY MUNCHIE (OPTIONAL): raw vegetable salad with no-oil salad dressing

ADDED FAT (OPTIONAL): 1 teaspoon butter or margarine OR 1 teaspoon olive oil or canola oil OR 2 tablespoons sour cream OR 1 tablespoon salad dressing

Evening snack

Repeat earlier snack choices OR any power snack (pg. 19) OR 1 cup cereal with 1 cup skim milk

Free items

raw vegetables, mustard, vinegar, lemon juice, no-oil salad dressing

16

Beautiful Foods for Beautiful Bodies and Babies

Nothing keeps a mother's feet on the ground
like having a little responsibility placed on
her shoulders.

There are certain foods that carry a powerful punch! They're
loaded with the vitamins and minerals you and your sweet
baby need to be healthy.

Get more of these into your grocery cart and your diet, and you'll
see a big difference in your energy, stamina, hair, skin, nails, and
general well-being right away. Looking good and feeling good come
from the inside. One day your baby will arise and call you blessed!

The Ten Best Foods

1. *Broccoli.* This is the best one-stop vegetable for beta
   carotene, fiber, and vitamins C, A, and folic acid. It also
   contains sulforaphane, which blocks cancer growth.

2. *Chicken or turkey.* These low-fat meats are packed with
   protein, iron, and zinc and are great choices for building
   your baby and your body. Cook them in lean, flavorful
   ways.

3. *Fish.* These are loaded with the valuable oils that provide protection and building of your baby's intelligence.

4. *Legumes (dried beans and peanuts).* These high-fiber

beauties are high in protein and complex carbohydrates, along with phytochemicals, bioflavonoids, calcium, and magnesium.

5. *Oranges.* This citrus fruit is a great source of vitamin C and, along with mangoes, a rich source of bioflavonoids that power our immune systems.

6. *Sweet potatoes.* Just one of these every day provides enough beta carotene to protect and build your baby and body.

7. *Skim or low-fat dairy products.* Milk, cheeses, and yogurts are loaded with calcium and magnesium that keep your blood pressure more stable and build your baby's skeletal system while keeping yours strong and intact. They're also excellent low-fat sources of protein.

8. *Spinach.* This dark green leafy provides a bumper crop of vitamins A and C along with folic acid. It also gives you valuable magnesium.

9. *Strawberries and tomatoes.* These red beauties are rich in substances that bolster your and your baby's immunities.

10. *Whole grains—breads, cereals, crackers, rice, pasta.* Loaded with B vitamins, selenium, magnesium, and vitamin E, these foods enhance the immunities and stabilize blood chemistries to boost mood, energy, and stress resiliency.

The Ten Worst Foods

1. *Artificial fruit drinks*—nothing more than sugar and water with artificial flavor and coloring added.

2. *Smoked or cured meats*—bacon, corned beef, ham, pastrami, and sausage. These are loaded with saturated fats, salt, and preservatives.

3. *Breakfast or granola bars*—candy bars rolled in oats! Loaded with sugar and fat.

4. *Chocolate*—high in saturated fat, caffeine, and sugar.

5. *Donuts*—white flour and sugar fried in animal fat.

6. *Processed meats*—hot dogs, bologna, and salami. These are high in saturated fat, salt, and preservatives that have been linked to cancer.

7. *Liver*—high in iron as it may be, it is an animal's filter that collects insecticides, poisons, and cholesterol.

8. *Snack chips and French fries*—triple threats: high in saturated fats, salt, and calories.

9. *Sodas*—most have twelve teaspoons sugar per can.

10. *Nondairy creamer or whipped topping*—a chemical nonfood comprised of hydrogenated fats and sugar.

HEALTHY GOAL: LEARN THE TEN BEST AND TEN WORST FOODS. INCREASE YOUR INTAKE OF THE BEST, DECREASE OR ELIMINATE YOUR INTAKE OF THE WORST, AND SEE HOW MUCH BETTER YOU FEEL AND LOOK!

Survival Planning for Quick Meals

This is for the people with the philosophy, "If it takes longer to cook it than to eat it, *forget it!*" There are few pregnant moms with the time or inclination to spend all afternoon preparing the dinner meal. Actually, lack of time can be a major obstacle to a wellness strategy.

Timesaving Strategies

- When you cook, do so in abundance, and then freeze properly portioned leftovers in freezer bags. This will provide quick meals when you need them.
- Keep two empty storage boxes (shoe boxes will do) in your freezer to store ready-made meals. Put main-dish portions in one box, complements to the meal (rice, pasta, vegetables) in the other.
- Spend just one hour on a weekend putting together some of the basics that will make each night's meal a healthy delight with a minimum of effort. For example, cook a big pot of brown rice or whole-wheat pasta; it can be heated during the week as needed. Or measure it out in servings, freeze in freezer bags, and reheat in the microwave or boiling water. Make a big batch of tomato sauce for use with pasta or as a topping for meat or pita pizzas. Cook a

pot of beans for beans and rice or bean quesadillas or burritos.

- For extra quick stir-fry, use frozen bags of assorted vegetable mixes. The vegetables are already cut, and they can be fully cooked in four minutes! Bags of frozen peas can also be used for a quick complex carbohydrate.
- For basic quick salads, tear romaine lettuce and top with a tomato, a no-oil Italian dressing, and a sprinkle of Parmesan.
- Prepare the marinade for Hawaiian Chicken; marinate enough boneless chicken breasts for two meals—half can be sliced and used in stir-fry with vegetables one night; the other breasts can be put on the grill.
- Cut up a plastic bag full of various vegetables: zucchini, broccoli, cauliflower, mushrooms, and carrots. Part may be marinated in low-calorie Italian dressing for a quick salad, or simply add a can of tuna to make a main dish and cooked pasta to make a great meal. The remaining vegetables may be used to steam or stir-fry.
- Sliced melon, fresh pineapple, or strawberries are a refreshing and quick complement to any meal!

A Week of Fast and Fabulous Dinners

Monday:

Grilled Marinated Chicken Breast
Brown Rice
Steamed Vegetables
Romaine Lettuce Salad With Sliced Oranges

Tuesday:

Whole-Wheat Pasta Topped With
    Tomato Sauce and Grated Mozarella Cheese
Steamed Broccoli
Marinated Vegetables
Fresh Fruit Medley Topped With Yogurt

Wednesday:

Stir-Fried Vegetables and Chicken Tossed With Pasta
Romaine Lettuce Salad With Tomatoes

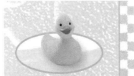

Items to Keep on Hand:

◦ Cooked angel-hair pasta (cook al dente, drain, and toss very lightly with olive oil; store in gallon Ziploc bags)

◦ Marinated, grilled breasts of chicken (store in Ziploc bags in freezer)

◦ Classico Tomato & Basil Sauce

◦ Bags of finely shredded fat-free or part-skim cheddar cheese or feta cheese

◦ Bags of salad greens

◦ Low-fat vinaigrettes

◦ Baking potatoes

◦ Smoked turkey breast and canned white meat chicken

◦ Canned chicken stock

◦ Canned whole tomatoes

◦ Canned beans: black, white cannelini, ranch beans

Thursday:

Beans Over Brown Rice With Grated Cheese
Steamed Vegetables
Fresh Fruit

Friday:

Grilled Chicken on Whole-Wheat Bun
Lettuce and Tomato Slices
Marinated Vegetable Salad

Saturday:

GO OUT TO EAT (or use up any leftovers)

Sunday:

Bean Burritos
Sliced Melon

My Quickest Meals

1. *Cheese Quesadillas:* Fat-free tortillas sprinkled with shredded part-skim cheddar cheese and drizzled with salsa—folded and browned in non-stick skillet till cheese melts. Serve with apple slices.

2. *Baked Spaghetti:* Cooked angel-hair pasta in a sheet pan—topped with one jar of Classico Tomato & Basil Sauce and sprinkled with one pound shredded mozzarella cheese. Bake for eight to ten minutes at 375 degrees. Serve with "Salad in a Bag" and a low-fat vinaigrette dressing.

3. *Vegetable Tortilla Pizza:* Large flour tortilla brushed with Classico's Tomato & Basil Sauce, topped with chopped veggies of choice, and sprinkled with grated mozzarella. Bake until lightly browned and crisp

(about five minutes) at 450 degrees. (See recipe on page 132.) Serve with baby carrots for munchies.

4. *Grilled Chicken Sandwich:* Grilled, marinated chicken breast (from your freezer) on whole-grain bun with lettuce, tomato, salsa, or Dijon mustard. Serve with fresh fruit.

5. *Smoked Turkey and White Bean Soup:* Smoked turkey breast (precooked) made into soup with chicken stock and cannelini beans. (See recipe on page 131.) Serve with raw veggies and fruit.

6. *Quick Taco Salad:* Canned black beans (rinsed) spiced with creole seasoning and sprinkled with shredded part-skim cheddar cheese. Heat and serve over mixed greens and crumbled Baked Tostitos with salsa. Serve with sliced oranges.

7. *Even Quicker Greek Salad:* Mixed greens (from a bag) topped with crumbled feta cheese, shredded Healthy Choice ham, and drizzled with low-fat vinaigrette. Serve with toasted petite pita and a piece of fruit.

8. *Cheese Baked Potatoes:* Microwave potatoes for four minutes each—cut open and top with cooked broccoli florets and Laughing Cow cheese wedges (two per potato) or part-skim-milk cheese. Microwave again until cheese melts. Top with nonfat sour cream. Serve with salad and low-fat vinaigrette.

17

Healthy Expectations
for Dining Out

ASK YOUR CHILD WHAT HE WANTS FOR DINNER ONLY IF
HE'S BUYING.

—Fran Lebowitz

 New research shows that America spends 40 percent of its food dollars dining away from home; dining out is no longer just for special occasions. For the health-conscious, dining out presents a culinary challenge: to enjoy fine food without compromising health.

The health dangers of dining out lie mostly in the hidden fats; the typical restaurant meal will give the equivalent of twelve to fourteen pats of butter! Never be timid about ordering foods in a special style. You are paying (and paying well!) for the meal and the service, and you deserve to have foods prepared to your preference. Learn to be discriminating, not intimidated!

A Discriminating Guide

Plan ahead. When you're in charge, choose a restaurant that you know and trust for quality food and a willingness to prepare foods in a healthful way upon request. More and more restaurants recognize that this trend toward healthy eating is not a passing fad; many progressive and responsible restaurants have begun to offer healthy menu selections. Supporting these restaurants will help to establish this tremendous service to the discerning diner.

Read between the lines. Think before you order. Menus are filled with clues about what the selections contain. Avoid these words:

- à la mode (with ice cream)
- au fromage (with cheese)
- au gratin (in cheese sauce)
- au lait (with milk)
- basted (with extra fat)
- bisque (cream soup)
- buttered (with extra fat)
- casserole (in some type of cream sauce)
- creamed (in extra fat)
- crispy (fried)
- escalloped (with cream sauce)
- hash (with extra fat)
- hollandaise (with cream sauce)
- pan-fried (in fat)
- sautéed (fried with extra fat)

If you see these words in the description of an appealing entrée, be bold enough to ask for the entrée prepared in a special way. If the description says "buttered," ask for it without the added butter. If the description says "pan-fried," ask for it grilled or poached instead. Entrées poached in wine or lemon juice are good choices, as are those simmered in tomato sauce. A baked potato or a side of pasta with red sauce is often a better choice than rice pilaf, which is prepared in oil.

Ask questions. Remember—it's your health, your money, and your waistline. If you have concerns about the way something will be prepared, discuss it kindly with the server. Don't be intimidated by the server or the people with whom you are eating.

Make special requests. Learn to say "on the side" and "no butter." Even though not stated on the menu, most foods will be prepared with fat, and more will be added before it is served to you. Ask for your salad dressing "on the side" (then apply sparingly; add extra lemon juice or vinegar for moistness). Order meats, fish, or poultry broiled or grilled without butter and with sauces on the side. When fresh vegetables are available, ask for them steamed without butter. If you order a baked potato, ask for it without butter or sour cream; request salsa, cottage cheese, grated Parmesan, or mustard to the side.

Monitor extra fats. Watch for the pats of butter, the cream in coffee, and the whipped cream on desserts. If the restaurant brings bread and rolls to the table, ask them to remove the butter (if no one in your party objects!). It's too easy to find yourself spreading that roll liberally with butter. Good crusty rolls really don't need the extra fat, especially when they are heated. The heat brings out natural flavor and makes them more satisfying. When the dessert tray comes by, ask for fresh berries (a much healthier choice than mousse).

Controlling Portions

As an adult there are no rewards for cleaning your plate. Restaurant portions can be huge, yet we often eat them. Many restaurants are answering the cry of "too much" by offering luncheon options at dinnertime. You do have other choices: Smaller appetizer selections are often just right and make a fine meal with an à la carte salad.

Try ordering one meal (and an extra plate) to share. And don't forget "take home." You can enjoy what's left as an elegant lunch the next day.

Never eat "all you can eat" at brunches, buffets, or covered-dish dinners—affairs that can easily become feeding frenzies! Instead, revise your perspective from "I need to get my money's worth" to "Look at all I have to choose from."

Healthful Dining Strategies

Let's look at the good and bad qualities of various cuisines and restaurants. Think about this information as you consider the "healthy expectations choices" when eating away from home.

Breakfast Out:

If you buy breakfast later than usual, eat a snack when you first get up to gear up your metabolism and begin to stabilize your body.

Order unbuttered whole-wheat toast, then add one teaspoon of butter, if desired. Grits may be substituted for a serving of bread, but be sure to order them unbuttered.

It's usually safer to order à la carte so you are not paying for, or being tempted by, the abundance of unhealthy food in the "breakfast specials" or buffets.

Be bold and creative. Rather than accepting French toast with syrup and bacon, ask for it prepared with whole-wheat bread, no syrup, and a side dish of fresh berries or fruit. Many restaurants will substitute cottage cheese or an egg for the breakfast meat.

Many restaurants serve oatmeal and cereal even though it's not on the menu. It's a nice whole-grain carbohydrate. Don't forget to ask for low-fat milk or yogurt, and top it with fresh berries or a banana.

Always look for a protein and a carbohydrate—more than a Danish!

Healthy Choices:
- cereal with skim milk and fruit
- French toast (with whole-wheat bread) and berries
- fresh fruit with cottage cheese or yogurt and whole-wheat toast
- fresh vegetable egg-white omelet and toast
- scrambled egg substitute and unbuttered whole-wheat toast

Dining Out:

Italian

Portion control is very important here. Although pasta with red sauce is a relatively low-fat choice, a plateful is five times too much! Order a side portion or an appetizer serving of pasta with steamed seafood or grilled chicken or fish.

Alfredo sauce is deadly, as is any white sauce. Ask for red sauce substitution.

Garlic bread sticks are rolled in butter, then garlic. Special order without butter, and you'll receive them straight from the oven!

Warning words: Alfredo, cheese sauce, cream sauce, fried, pancetta, parmigiana, prosciutto, saltimbocca, white sauce.

Healthy Choices:
- cioppino (seafood soup) or minestrone
- clams, mussels, or scallops linguine with red sauce
- grilled chicken with pasta marinara
- grilled fresh fish with pasta marinara
- pasta e fagioli and salad

Mexican

Ask that your salad be brought in place of the chips. It will help stop the munch-a-bunch syndrome.

Order à la carte; whole meal selections are laden with high-fat side dishes, such as refried beans (often made with pure lard).

Ask that the sour cream and cheese be omitted from your dish. The cheese is a high-fat cheese with ten grams of fat per ounce.

Ask for guacamole on the side; two tablespoons contain the fat of a pat of butter.

Never, never eat the fried tortilla shells that contain Mexican salads. Think of them as inedible, hard plastic bowls. They are sponges for the grease they are cooked in.

Warning words: chimichangas, chorizo, con queso, fried, guacamole, served in a tortilla shell, shredded cheese, sour cream, tortilla chips.

Healthy Choices:
- black bean soup or gazpacho
- chicken burrito or tostada
- chicken enchiladas
- chicken fajitas (without added fat)
- chili with salad
- soft chicken tacos

Oriental

Chinese, Korean, Thai, or Vietnamese food is an excellent choice for dining out, as stir-frying is the main method of cooking. This terrific technique cooks the vegetables quickly, retaining the nutrients and using very little oil.

Order dishes lightly stir-fried (not deep-fried like egg rolls) and without heavy gravies or sweet-and-sour sauces.

Half-a-dinner portion is appropriate, with steamed brown or white rice. (Fried rice is just that—fried!)

Ask for food prepared *without* MSG, and be careful with the soy sauce you add. (Both are loaded with sodium!)

This is not the time to order sushi, even at highly reputable restaurants that serve the freshest fish from the best sources. Have grilled teriyaki fish instead.

Warning words: deep-fried, battered, fried, crispy, cashews, fried noodles, duck, bird's nest, tempura, tonkatsu (fried pork), torikatsu (fried chicken).

Healthy Choices:
- bamboo-steamed vegetables with scallops, chicken, or whole steamed fish
- moo goo gai pan (no MSG, little oil)
- tofu with vegetables (no MSG, little oil)
- udon (noodles) served with meat and vegetables
- wonton, hot and sour, or miso soup
- yakitori (meats broiled on skewers)

Seafood

Order fresh seafood when possible—steamed, boiled, grilled, or broiled without butter. For dipping, a small amount of cocktail sauce is a better choice than butter (two dips in butter equal fifty calories). When fried, small seafood items such as shrimp and oysters are deadly in terms of fat and calories; the surface area is high, more breading adheres, absorbing more fat. All seafood can be low-fat and low-sodium if grilled without butter and served without sauces.

Healthy Choices:
- fresh fish of the day (grilled or poached, without butter, sauce to the side)
- lobster, crab meat, crab claws
- mesquite-grilled shrimp
- scallops (grilled or broiled without butter)
- seafood kabobs (grilled without butter)
- steamed clams, mussels, oysters, or shrimp

Steak Houses

As with Italian restaurants, portion control is the key here. A sixteen-ounce steak or prime rib will give you five times more protein than needed. Order the smallest cut available (often a petite-cut fillet), and don't hesitate to take some home! You may do well to cut off an appropriate portion and separate it from the other on your plate. (Try this before you begin to eat, when control is at its highest!)

Remember always to have a complex carbohydrate and a protein source, never just meat and salad alone. Your carbohydrate may be a roll, a side of pasta, or a baked potato.

Healthy Choices:
- charbroiled shrimp (grilled without butter)
- Hawaiian or marinated grilled chicken breast
- petite-cut fillet
- shish kebab or brochette (grilled without butter)
- slices of London broil (no sauces or gravies)

Fast-Food Restaurants

Just say *no* to sauces: It's the mayonnaise, special sauces, and sour cream that triple the fat, sodium, and calories in fast foods; always order your food without them! And undress your salad; a single packet of regular dressing can contain as much fat as a double cheeseburger.

Shun the cheese. The varieties commonly used by the fast-food chains are high in fat, cholesterol, and calories.

Stuffed potatoes may seem a healthy addition to the fast-food menu, but not with the cheese sauces they hold—often the equivalent to nine pats of butter per potato! Try chili or broccoli and salsa instead.

Chicken is a lower-fat alternative to beef, but not when it's batter-fried. One serving of chicken nuggets has twice the fat of a regular hamburger. A chicken sandwich is no health package either. This greasy sandwich has enough fat to equal eleven pats of butter. The new grilled chicken sandwiches are much better, as long as you order them without the dressing and sauces.

Salad bars are a good way to add fiber and nutrients, but only the salad vegetables do so. Leave the mayonnaise-based salads, croutons, and bacon bits on the bar. Add extra lemon juice or vinegar for moistness.

Croissant sandwiches aren't a whole lot more than breakfast on a grease bun. Most croissants have the fat equivalent of more than four-and-one-half pats of butter, and the toppings add insult to injury!

Frozen yogurt, although lower in fat and cholesterol, contains more sugar than ice cream. It is not a perfectly healthy substitute.

Don't get discouraged and think you can't ever eat fast food and still be healthy. You can still have a healthy fast-food meal; the goal is to learn to make wise choices. Learn what and how to order fast food. Here is a guide to help you:

Burger King

Healthiest Choices:
- B.K. Broiler Chicken Sandwich (without ranch dressing or mayo)
- Hamburger Deluxe (no mayo)—for women
- Whopper (no mayo)—for men
- BK Broiler (with sauce it gives twenty-six grams of fat!)
- Chunky Chicken Salad with Newman's Own Reduced-Calorie Italian Dressing and crackers

You may order a side salad with any of the above meals (with the light Italian dressing). Some Burger King restaurants have also begun to offer fresh fruit.

Less is less. Although no burger is truly lean, the smaller the portion, the less fat you get. A Whopper Jr. without mayo, although filling and tasty, gives twenty-eight less grams of fat than the Big King.

Worst Choices:
- Breakfast or Burger Buddies
- Chicken Sandwich
- Croissan'wich with sausage, egg, and cheese
- Double Whopper with cheese
- Scrambled Egg Platter with sausage
- Big King

Chick-Fil-A

Healthiest Choices:
- Hearty Breast of Chicken Soup
- Chargrilled Chicken Salad (no-oil salad dressing)
- Chargrilled Chicken Sandwich (no mayo)

Worst Choices:
- All else

McDonald's

Healthiest Choices:
- McGrilled Chicken Classic (with BBQ sauce)
- Chunky Chicken Salad (with your own crackers for carbohydrate)
- Hamburger (small)
- McLean Deluxe Sandwich (no mayo)

Worst Choices:
- Big Mac
- Chicken McNuggets
- Arch Deluxe
- Quarter Pounder with cheese
- Sausage Biscuit with egg
- Sausage McMuffin with egg

Wendy's

Healthiest Choices:
- Baked Potato (plain, without cheese sauce, with a small chili)
- Grilled Chicken Sandwich (without honey mustard; it's in a fat base—try BBQ sauce for flavor)
- Grilled Chicken Salad with reduced-fat Italian dressing
- Single Hamburger (without mayo)
- Salad Bar (use raw vegetables as desired; avoid potato salad, macaroni salad, and the like; use garbanzo beans or chili for protein) with reduced-fat Italian dressing

Worst Choices:
- Big Bacon Classic
- Big Classic
- Crispy Chicken Nuggets
- Fish Fillet Sandwich
- Hot Stuffed Baked Potato
- Jr. Swiss Deluxe
- Pasta with Alfredo Sauce

Hardee's

Healthiest Choices:
- Chicken 'n' Pasta Salad
- Grilled Chicken Sandwich (no mayo)
- Hamburger (no mayo)

Worst Choices:
- Bacon Cheeseburger
- Big Country Breakfast with sausage or ham
- Big Deluxe Burger
- Fisherman's Fillet
- The Lean 1 (18 grams of fat!)

- Mushroom 'n' Swiss Burger

Taco Bell

Healthiest Choices:
- Light Taco Salad (skip the nacho chips)
- Light Chicken Burrito
- Light Chicken Soft Taco Supreme
- Light Bean Burrito

Worst Choices:
- Mexican Pizza
- Nachos BellGrande, Nachos Supreme
- Soft Taco Supreme
- Taco BellGrande
- Regular Taco Salad (61 grams of fat—905 calories!)

Arby's or Rax

Healthiest Choices:
- Arby's Grilled Chicken BBQ Sandwich (no mayo)
- Light Rax Turkey Delight (no mayo)
- Rax Turkey (no mayo)
- Roast Beef Sandwich (no sauce!)

Pizza Places

Healthiest Choices:
- personal-sized cheese pizza, with vegetables if desired (eat three-quarters and save the remaining quarter for a snack)
- thin-crust 13-inch (medium) cheese pizza, with vegetables (no sausage or pepperoni): two slices for women; three slices for men

Worst Choices:
- thick-crust or deep-dish pizza with sausage or pepperoni

Sub Shops or Delis

Healthiest Choices:
- mini-sub (turkey, roast beef; no oil or mayo)
- 6-inch sub (turkey, roast beef, cheese; no oil or mayo)
- veggie bar and turkey club
- Subway's Roasted Chicken on whole wheat (no mayo or dressing)

Worst Choices:
- tuna subs—loaded with fat

Deli and grocery stores will usually make you turkey, roast beef, or Jarlsberg Lite sandwiches (ask for three ounces of meat on sandwich).

Boston Market

Healthiest Choices:
- Turkey Breast Sandwich and Fruit Salad

Worst Choices:
- Boston Carver Chicken Sandwich (thirty-two grams of fat!)
- all else

Health or Natural Food Restaurants

Here you have an opportunity to get whole grains and fresh vegetable salads, but the fats and sodium can still sneak in quite deceptively. Beware of sauces and high-fat cheeses smothering the foods and high-fat dressings on salads and sandwiches. Many foods are prepared as they would be at a fast-food restaurant—but with healthier-sounding names.

The salads and salad bars may be lovely, but follow the guideline of dressing to the side, used sparingly. Many salad bars have a protein source in cottage cheese, grated cheese, or chopped eggs (aim for the egg whites, not the yolk).

If you have a cheese dish, use no other added fats. Ask if they can use mozzarella cheese (it is almost always partly skimmed of fat).

Healthiest Choices:
- bean soup with salad (dressing on side)
- chef-type salad with whole-grain roll (no ham or cheese)
- fruit plate with nonfat plain yogurt or cottage cheese and whole-grain roll
- pita stuffed with vegetables and meat or mozzarella cheese
- stir-fry dish (ask for "light on the soy sauce")

Part 3

RECIPES FOR A HEALTHY PREGNANCY

18

YOUR GROCERY LIST
FOR HEALTH

Take a long, hard look at your grocery cart. If it's a grease trap loaded with bacon, chips, and Twinkies, chances are you haven't been fixing the healthiest foods. Now is a good time to strengthen and streamline your food shopping, your fridge, and your home-cooked meals. Here are some quick tips for adding a health advantage to your shopping cart:

BUYING THE BASICS

Whole grain is a must for fiber and nutrition. The word *whole* should be the first word of the ingredient list, such as "whole wheat, whole oats." Also check labels for hidden fats and hidden sugars; some cereals, like granola, are nutritional nightmares in a bowl. Remember the available variety of whole-grain English muffins, bagels, pita breads and, of course, rice cakes. Stock up on whole-wheat or artichoke pastas and brown rice. Incorporate barley, oats, cracked wheat and cornmeal into recipes. Include dried or canned beans, split peas, lentils, and chickpeas.

Daring Dairy

Although they get a bad rap these days, dairy foods are a treasure chest of protein, calcium, and other body-building nutrients. But they can also be loaded with fat, so look for lower-fat variations on favorites: skim milk, buttermilk, nonfat yogurt, skim milk ricotta, pot or farmer's cheese, part-skim mozzarella, and skim milk cottage cheese. Check the labels to be sure they fit your nutrition standards of having fewer than three grams of fat per hundred-calorie serving.

Doing the Deli

Select sliced turkey or chicken, lean ham, and low-fat cheeses instead of the usual lunch meats. Limit use of high-fat, high-sodium processed sausages and meats, hot dogs, bacon, and salami.

Fending Against Fats and Oils

Limit use of butter, margarines, and cream cheese. Select reduced-fat or light mayonnaises and salad dressings. Do not use polyunsaturated oils, but instead use olive or canola oil in small amounts. All of these choices should be used sparingly. Remember that it's the fat that makes you unhealthy, fat, and slows you down!

Making Meat Choices

All cuts should be lean and trimmed of visible fat. Choose the following: beef—round, loin, sirloin, and extra lean ground beef; lamb—leg, arm, loin, rib; pork—tenderloin, leg, shoulder; turkey or chicken—skinless; fish and shellfish—fresh, just delivered.

Water, Water Everywhere

Stock up on bottled waters to replace sugary sodas, which offer zero nutrition and lots of calories. Try sparkling mineral waters (add a splash of fruit juice for flavor).

Picking Produce

Fruits and vegetables are no-fat, no-cholesterol beauties with fiber that help in stabilizing the body—providing for lower cholesterol levels, boosted immunities against sicknesses, lovelier skin, nails, and hair, higher energy levels, and less body aches and pains. Keep enough on hand so that you can always make a salad. Buy the freshest—and the most colorful—produce possible for top nutrition.

Generally, the more vivid the coloring of the pulp, the more essential nutrients it holds.

Wonderfully fresh fruits and vegetables are a particular passion of mine. For the sweetest produce, choose what is in season—a good price and abundant supply will tell you a fruit or vegetable is at its peak. Ask at your grocery store or farmer's market which are freshest buying days and where the vegetables are grown; search for locally grown and in-season fruits and vegetables. Out-of-season produce is more expensive and often imported. If it is imported, it may be only spot-checked for pesticide residues. (Use the fruit and vegetable guide on pages 39–41 when getting ready to purchase fruit or vegetables.)

When fresh is not possible, frozen is the next choice; avoid vegetables that are prepared with butters or sauces and fruits that are packed with sugar. (Freezing foods doesn't destroy their nutrients and quality as readily as canning does.)

Take advantage of your grocer's pre-cut, pre-chopped vegetables and fruits. They are available in the produce area or may be purchased by the pound from the salad bar.

GRAINS AND BREADS
Brown rice: ❑ Instant
  ❑ Long-grain
  ❑ Short-grain
  ❑ Wild rice
  ❑ Arborio rice
  ❑ Cornmeal
  ❑ Couscous
Tortillas, flour:
  ❑ Mission
  ❑ Buena Vida Fat-Free
❑ Whole-wheat bagels
❑ 100% whole-wheat bread
("whole" is the first word of the ingredients)
❑ Whole-wheat English muffins
❑ Whole-wheat hamburger buns
Whole-wheat or artichoke pasta:
  ❑ Angel hair
  ❑ Elbows
  ❑ Flat
  ❑ Lasagna ❑ Orzo
  ❑ Penne ❑ Spaghetti
  ❑ Rotini *(spirals)*
❑ Whole-wheat pastry flour
❑ Whole-wheat pita bread
❑ _____
CEREALS *(whole grain and less than 5 grams of added sugar)*:
❑ All Bran With Extra Fiber

❑ Cheerios
❑ Familia Müesli
❑ Granola
❑ Grape-Nuts
❑ Grits ❑ Kashi
❑ Kellogg's Just Right
❑ Kellogg's Low-Fat Granola
❑ Kellogg's Nutri-Grain Almond Raisin
❑ Kellogg's Raisin Squares
❑ Nabisco Shredded Wheat
❑ Ralston Müesli
Oats: ❑ Old-fashioned
  ❑ Quick-cooking
❑ Post Bran Flakes
Puffed cereals: ❑ Rice
  ❑ Wheat
  ❑ Shredded Wheat 'N' Bran
Unprocessed bran:
  ❑ Oat
  ❑ Wheat
❑ Wheatena
❑ _____
CRACKERS
Crispbread: ❑ Kavli
  ❑ Wasa
  ❑ Crispy cakes
❑ Health Valley graham crackers
❑ Harvest Crisps 5-Grain
❑ Mr. Phipps Rice Cakes: ❑ Plain
❑ Quaker Banana Nut
❑ Ry Krisp
❑ _____

DAIRY
❑ Butter ❑ Light butter
Cheese *(low-fat—fewer than 5 grams of fat per ounce)*:
Cheddar:
  ❑ Kraft Fat-Free
  ❑ Kraft Natural Reduced Fat
  ❑ Cottage cheese *(1% or nonfat)*
Cream cheese:
  ❑ Philadelphia Light *(tub)*
  ❑ Philadelphia Free
  ❑ Farmer's
  ❑ Jarlsberg Lite
Mozzarella: ❑ Nonfat
  ❑ Part-skim
  ❑ String cheese
Nonrefrigerated:
  ❑ Laughing Cow Light
  ❑ Parmesan
Ricotta: ❑ Nonfat
  ❑ Skim milk
  ❑ Sun-Ni Armenian String
❑ Egg substitute
❑ Eggs
❑ Milk *(skim or 1%)*
❑ Nonfat sour cream
❑ Nonfat plain yogurt
❑ Stonyfield Farm yogurt
❑ _____
CANNED GOODS
Chicken broth:
  ❑ Swanson's
  ❑ Natural Goodness
❑ Evaporated skim milk

❑ Hearts of Palm
Soups:
  ❑ Healthy Choice
  ❑ Pritikin
  Progresso:
    ❑ Hearty Black Bean
    ❑ Lentil
Tomatoes:
  ❑ Paste ❑ Sauce
  ❑ Stewed ❑ Whole
❑ _____

CONDIMENTS
❑ Honey
Hot Pepper Sauce:
  ❑ Pickapeppa sauce
  ❑ Shriracha Chili
    Sauce
  ❑ Jamaican Hell Fire
  ❑ Tabasco
Mayonnaise:
  ❑ Light
  ❑ Miracle Whip
    Light
Mustard:
  ❑ Dijon ❑ Spicy hot
❑ Pepperoncini peppers
Salad Dressing:
  ❑ Bernstein's
Reduced Calorie
  ❑ Good Seasons
  ❑ Kraft Free
  ❑ Jardine's Fat-Free
    Garlic
  ❑ Vinaigrette
  ❑ Pritikin
❑ Soy sauce *(low-sodium)*
❑ Salsa or picante sauce
Spices and herbs:
  ❑ Allspice
  ❑ Basil

❑ Black pepper
❑ Cayenne
❑ Celery seed
❑ Chili powder
❑ Cinnamon
❑ Creole seasoning
❑ Curry
❑ Dill weed
❑ Five spice
❑ Garlic powder
❑ Ginger
❑ Mrs. Dash
  Original Blend
❑ Mrs. Dash Garlic
  and Herb
Seasoning:
  ❑ Mustard
  ❑ Nutmeg
  ❑ Oregano
  ❑ Onion powder
  ❑ Paprika ❑ Parsley
  ❑ Pepper, cracked
  ❑ Rosemary
  ❑ Saffron
  ❑ Salt ❑ Thyme
Fresh herbs:
  ❑ Basil
  ❑ Chives ❑ Cilantro
  ❑ Ginger ❑ Parsley
  ❑ Rosemary
  ❑ Thyme
❑ Vanilla extract
Vinegars:
  ❑ Balsamic
  ❑ Cider
  ❑ Red wine
  ❑ Rice wine
  ❑ Tarragon
  ❑ White wine
❑ White Wine

❑ Worcestershire sauce
❑ _____

FRUITS
Fresh fruits:
  ❑ Apples ❑ Apricots
  ❑ Bananas ❑ Berries
  ❑ Cherries
  ❑ Dates *(unsweetened, pitted)*
  ❑ Grapefruit
  ❑ Grapes ❑ Kiwi
  ❑ Lemons ❑ Limes
  ❑ Mango ❑ Melon
  ❑ Nectarines
  ❑ Oranges ❑ Papaya
  ❑ Peaches ❑ Pears
  ❑ Pineapple
  ❑ Plantains
  ❑ Plums
Dried fruits:
  ❑ Apricots
  ❑ Peaches
  ❑ Pineapple
  ❑ Raisins (dark and
    golden)
❑ Mixed
❑ _____

VEGETABLES
❑ Asparagus ❑ Beets
❑ Bell peppers
❑ Broccoli
❑ Brussels sprouts
❑ Cabbage
❑ Carrots
❑ Cauliflower ❑ Celery
❑ Corn
❑ Cucumbers
❑ Eggplant
❑ Garlic ❑ Green beans
❑ Greens

❏ Hot peppers ❏ Kale
❏ Mushrooms ❏ Okra
❏ Onions ❏ Peas
❏ Red potatoes
❏ Radicchio
❏ Romaine lettuce
❏ Salad greens
❏ Shallots
❏ Simply Potatoes hash browns
❏ Spinach
❏ Squash *(yellow, crook neck)*
❏ Sugar snap peas *(frozen)*
❏ Sun-dried tomatoes
❏ Sweet potatoes
❏ Tomatoes
❏ White potatoes
❏ Zucchini
❏ _____

BEANS AND MEATS

Beans and peas:
❏ Black
❏ Chickpeas/ garbanzo beans
❏ Cannelini
❏ Kidney ❏ Lentils
❏ Navy ❏ Pinto
❏ Split peas
❏ _____

Beef *(lean)*:
❏ Deli-sliced
❏ Ground round
❏ London broil
❏ Round steak
❏ _____

Fish and seafood:
❏ Clams
❏ Cod ❏ Grouper

❏ Mussels
❏ Salmon ❏ Scallops
❏ Shrimp ❏ Snapper
❏ Swordfish ❏ Tuna
❏ _____

Lamb:
❏ Leg ❏ Loin chops

Pork:
❏ Canadian bacon
❏ Center-cut chops
❏ Tenderloin

Chicken:
❏ Boneless breasts
❏ Legs/thighs
❏ Whole fryer

Turkey:
❏ Bacon ❏ Breast
❏ Ground
❏ Deli-sliced
❏ Whole
❏ _____

Veal:
❏ Chops ❏ Cutlets
❏ Ground

Water-packed cans:
❏ Chicken
❏ Salmon ❏ Tuna
❏ Charlie's Lunch Kit
❏ _____

MISCELLANEOUS

All-fruit spreads and pourable fruit:
❏ Knudsen
❏ Polaner
❏ Smucker's Simply Fruit
❏ Welch's Totally Fruit
❏ Baking powder

❏ Baking soda

Bean dips:
❏ Jardine's
❏ Guiltless Gourmet
❏ Bread crumbs

Cooking oils:
❏ Canola ❏ Olive
❏ Cornstarch

Fruit Juices *(unsweetened)*:
❏ Apple
❏ Cranberry-apple
❏ White grape
❏ Orange
❏ Nonstick cooking spray

Nuts/seeds *(dry-roasted, unsalted)*:
❏ Peanuts
❏ Sunflower kernels
❏ Pecans ❏ Walnuts

Pasta Sauce:
❏ Pritikin
❏ Classico Tomato & Basil
❏ Ragú Chunky Gardenstyle
❏ Peanut butter *(natural)*
❏ Phyllo dough

Popcorn: ❏ Orville Redenbacher's Natural Light or Smart Pop microwave popcorn
❏ Plain kernels

Tortilla chips:
❏ Baked Tostitos
❏ Guiltless Gourmet
❏ Water *(spring or sparkling)*

19

SUNNY BREAKFASTS

Remember—breakfast is the "stick" that stokes your metabolic fire. Don't resort to the food industry's versions of "instant" breakfasts, like toaster fruit pies, granola bars (just candy with oats), and artificially flavored and colored powdered drink mixes. Instead of going for breakfast in the fast lane—and getting much more fat, calories, and sodium than you've bargained for—grab and go with your own quick and easy breakfast. Your body will be grateful and will gladly return the favor by working for you rather than working against you.

You need more than just a piece of toast and coffee to give your baby a "sunny beginning." When you grab coffee and toast, you're depriving your body of the simple carbohydrates and protein it needs to get started. American breakfast favorites focus on the complex carbohydrates (bagels, English muffins, pancakes, muffins, and toast) but ignore the rest.

Try the following breakfast ideas, a different one every day, for a wonderful variety of ways to start your day just right!

Cheese Danish

1 whole-wheat English muffin
2 oz. light or nonfat cream cheese
2 Tbsp. raisins OR all-fruit preserves

Spread muffin with light or nonfat cream cheese; if possible, warm in toaster oven. Top with raisins or preserves. (Another marvelous choice: Mash ¹/₄ cup fresh berries and put on top of cheese and muffin.)

Makes 1 serving, giving 2 complex carbohydrates (muffin), 2 ounces protein (cheese), and 1 simple carbohydrate (raisins).

Nutritional profile per serving:
Using fat-free cream cheese:
48 g carbohydrate; 12 g protein; 1 g fat; 0% calories from fat; 10 mg cholesterol; 736 mg sodium; 249 calories
Using light cream cheese:
48 g carbohydrate; 12 g protein; 11 g fat; 30% calories from fat; 48 mg cholesterol; 736 mg sodium; 328 calories

Hot Apple-Cinnamon Oatmeal

²/₃ cup old-fashioned oats
1 cup skim milk
¹/₂ cup unsweetened apple or white grape juice
1 Tbsp. raisins
cinnamon
¹/₂ tsp. vanilla

Bring milk, apple juice, and oats to a boil. Gently cook for 5 minutes, stirring occasionally. Add raisins, vanilla, and cinnamon; let sit covered for 2–3 minutes to thicken. This recipe also cooks well in the microwave. Combine all ingredients and cook for 3 to 4 minutes on high.

Makes 1 serving, giving 2 complex carbohydrates (oats), 2 ounces protein (milk), and 1 simple carbohydrate (juice and raisins).

Nutritional profile per serving:
63 g carbohydrate; 17 g protein; 4 g fat; 10% calories from fat; 4 mg cholesterol; 131 mg sodium; 357 calories

Orange Vanilla French Toast

6 egg whites, lightly beaten
1 tsp. vanilla
$1^{1}/_{2}$ cups skim milk
$^{1}/_{2}$ tsp. cinnamon
6 slices whole-wheat bread
all-fruit preserves (no sugar) or mashed fresh fruit

NOTE: Add the juice of half an orange, and it's even better! You can freeze the extras and pop them in the toaster on a busy morning.

Beat together egg whites, milk, vanilla, and cinnamon. Add bread slices one at a time, letting the bread absorb liquid in the process. May let the bread sit for a few minutes. Spray nonstick skillet with cooking spray, and then heat. Gently lift the bread with spatula into skillet and cook until golden brown on each side. Serve topped with $^{1}/_{2}$ cup fresh fruit or 1 tablespoon (no sugar) all-fruit preserves.

Makes 3 servings, giving 2 complex carbohydrates (bread), 2 ounces protein (eggs, milk), and 1 simple carbohydrate (fruit).

Nutritional profile per serving:
55 g carbohydrate; 20 g protein; 3 g fat;
7% calories from fat; 3 mg cholesterol;
529 mg sodium; 329 calories

Peanut Butter Danish

2 slices 100% whole-grain bread
1 Tbsp. natural peanut butter
$^{1}/_{2}$ banana
8 oz. skim milk

Slice banana lengthwise and place with inside facing down on the slice of bread. Top with peanut butter. Broil until peanut butter is slightly brown and bubbly. Surprise! Have with an 8-ounce glass of skim milk.

Makes 1 serving, giving 2 complex carbohydrates (bread), protein (peanut butter and milk), and 1 simple carbohydrate (banana).

Nutritional profile per serving:
53 g carbohydrate; 18 g protein; 10 g fat;
25% calories from fat; 4 mg cholesterol;
418 mg sodium; 374 calories

Cheese Apple Surprise

2 slices whole-wheat bread
1 Tbsp. raisins
$1/2$ apple, thinly sliced
2 oz. mozzarella cheese

Top bread with apple and raisins. Place cheese on apple-raisin layer. Broil until cheese is bubbly.

Makes 1 serving, giving 2 complex carbohydrates (bread), 2 ounces protein (cheese), and 1 simple carbohydrate (apple and raisins).

Nutritional profile per serving:
41 g carbohydrate; 19 g protein; 11 g fat;
30% calories from fat; 32 mg cholesterol;
586 mg sodium; 332 calories

Breakfast Shake

$1/2$ cup frozen fruit*
1 cup skim milk
1 tsp. vanilla
2 Tbsp. nonfat dry milk
2 Tbsp. wheat germ
2 tsp. oat bran

Blend frozen fruit in blender. Add remaining ingredients and continue blending till smooth.

Makes 1 serving, giving 1 complex carbohydrate (wheat germ and bran), 2 ounces protein (milk), and 1 simple carbohydrate (fruit).

*Don't throw away your very ripe bananas. Peel and freeze in freezer bags and use for your shakes.

Nutritional profile per serving:
32 g carbohydrate; 16 g protein; 2 g fat;
10% calories from fat; 5 mg cholesterol;
176 mg sodium; 200 calories

Breakfast Sundae Supreme

$^{1}/_{2}$ banana, quartered lengthwise
$^{1}/_{2}$ cup nonfat ricotta cheese
$^{1}/_{4}$ cup strawberries, sliced
$^{1}/_{4}$ cup crushed pineapple, canned in own juice
2 Tbsp. Grape-Nuts or low-fat granola
1 tsp. honey or all-fruit pourable syrup

Place the banana quarters star-fashioned on a small plate. Scoop ricotta cheese onto the center points. Surround with the other fruit; then sprinkle with cereal. Drizzle with honey or all-fruit syrup.

Makes one serving, giving 1 complex carbohydrate (cereal), 2 ounces protein (ricotta), and 2 simple carbohydrates (fruit).

Nutritional profile per serving:
42 g carbohydrate; 15 g protein; 1 g fat;
4% calories from fat; 5 mg cholesterol;
111 mg sodium; 224 calories

Spiced Bran Muffin With Shake-'em-up Shake

Spiced Bran Muffins

$^{1}/_{4}$ cup molasses
3 Tbsp. honey
2 large egg whites
$^{1}/_{4}$ cup plain, nonfat yogurt
$^{1}/_{4}$ cup 1% or skim milk
$^{1}/_{4}$ cup wheat bran
$^{1}/_{4}$ cup oat bran
1 cup whole-wheat pastry flour
$1^{1}/_{2}$ tsp. baking powder
1 tsp. ground ginger
1 tsp. ground cloves
1 tsp. cinnamon
$^{1}/_{4}$ cup chopped pecans
$^{1}/_{4}$ cup golden raisins
nonstick cooking spray

Preheat oven to 350 degrees. Warm the molasses and honey in the microwave or in a saucepan until they just begin to steam (about 110 degrees). Let the mixture cool. Whisk the egg whites, yogurt, and milk together until blended. Add the molasses-honey mixture while whisking. Gently stir in the brans, flour, baking powder, and spices; then fold in the pecans and raisins.

Spray a 12-cup muffin tin with nonstick spray and fill each cup two-thirds full with batter. Bake for 15 to 20 minutes or until a toothpick inserted into the center of a muffin comes out clean. Serve warm, or freeze individually in freezer bags to use later.

Serve with a Shake-'em-up Shake.

Nutritional profile per muffin:
21 g carbohydrate; 3 g protein; 1.7 g fat;
15% calories from fat; 0 mg cholesterol;
28 mg sodium; 106 calories

Shake-'em-up Shake

8 oz. (1 cup) skim or 1% milk
$^{1}/_{2}$ cup fresh orange juice
1 tsp. vanilla
4 to 5 ice cubes

Pour all of the ingredients in a large cup with a lid. Shake wildly and drink up!
Serve with a spiced bran muffin.

Nutritional profile per serving:
25 g carbohydrate; 9 g protein; .6 g fat;
4% calories from fat; 4 mg cholesterol;
127 mg sodium; 142 calories

Baked Breakfast Apple

1 small Golden Delicious apple, cored
2 Tbsp. old-fashioned oats
$^{1}/_{4}$ tsp. cinnamon
1 Tbsp. raisins
2 Tbsp. apple juice
$^{1}/_{2}$ cup nonfat ricotta cheese

Place the apple in a microwaveable bowl. Mix together the oats, cinnamon, and raisins. Fill the cavity of the cored apple with the mixture. Pour the apple juice over the apple and cover it with plastic wrap. Microwave on high for 1 minute. Turn the dish around halfway and microwave for 1 minute more. Spoon the ricotta cheese onto a plate and top it with the apple and the heated juice mixture.

Makes 1 serving, giving 1 complex carbohydrate (oats), 2 ounces protein (ricotta), and 1 simple carbohydrate (apple, the juice, and the raisins).

Nutritional profile per serving:
30 g carbohydrate; 14 g protein; 1 g fat;
6% calories from fat; 23 mg cholesterol;
100 mg sodium; 183 calories

Scrambled Eggs Burrito

1 10-inch flour tortilla, preferably whole-wheat
$^1/_4$ tsp. creole seasoning
2 eggs, lightly beaten, or $^1/_2$ cup egg substitute
2 Tbsp. part-skim milk cheddar cheese, grated
$^1/_4$ cup picante sauce
nonstick cooking spray
$^1/_4$ cantaloupe, sliced

Heat a nonstick pan or griddle over medium high heat. Add the tortilla to heat and soften, turning it over after 15 seconds. After 15 seconds on the second side, remove the tortilla from the pan and wrap it in foil to keep warm. Spray the pan with nonstick spray, continuing to heat. Beat together the eggs, grated cheese, and creole seasoning. Add to the pan and scramble. Place the egg mixture on the tortilla and spoon on the picante sauce. Wrap it up burrito-style. Serve with the sliced cantaloupe.

Makes 1 serving, giving 1 complex carbohydrate (tortilla), 3 ounces protein (eggs and cheese), and 1 simple carbohydrate (cantaloupe).

Nutritional profile per serving:
32 g carbohydrate; 13 g protein; 5 g fat;
20% calories from fat (with egg substitute);
8 mg cholesterol; 613 mg sodium;
223 calories

Southwestern Fruit Toast

2 egg whites, lightly beaten
2 Tbsp. skim milk
$^1/_2$ tsp. vanilla
1 10-inch flour tortilla, preferably whole-wheat
nonstick cooking spray
2 Tbsp. low-fat granola
$^1/_2$ cup mixed berries
1 Tbsp. all-fruit syrup

Beat together the egg whites, milk, and vanilla. Dip the tortilla into the mixture, letting it absorb the liquid for a minute or so. Coat a nonstick skillet with nonstick spray, and then heat.

Gently lift the tortilla with a spatula, place it in the skillet, and cook until it is golden brown on each side. Sprinkle one-half of the tortilla with the granola and the fruit. Fold the tortilla over omelette-style and slide it onto a plate. Drizzle it with the all-fruit syrup.

Makes 1 serving, giving 2 complex carbohydrates (the tortilla and the granola), 2 ounces protein (the egg whites and the milk), and 2 simple carbohydrates (the fruit and fruit syrup).

Nutritional profile per serving:
44 g carbohydrate; 13.5 g protein; 2 g fat;
7% calories from fat; 8 mg cholesterol;
266 mg sodium; 249 calories

Hot Oatcakes

4 egg whites
1 cup nonfat ricotta cheese
2 Tbsp. canola oil
1 tsp. vanilla
$^2/_3$ cup old-fashioned oats, uncooked
$^1/_4$ tsp. salt
nonstick cooking spray
4 Tbsp. all-fruit jam or pourable all-fruit syrup

Measure the egg whites, cheese, oil, vanilla, oats, and salt into a blender or food processor and blend for 5 to 6 seconds. Spoon 2 tablespoons of the batter into a hot skillet sprayed with nonstick spray. Turn the pancakes when bubbles appear on the surface; cook them for 1 more minute.

For 1 serving, spread 3 pancakes with 1 tablespoon all-fruit jam or syrup. Makes 12 3-inch pancakes. Freeze the leftovers in individual freezer bags. When ready to use, toast the pancakes to thaw and heat.

Makes 4 servings, each giving 1 complex carbohydrate (pancakes), 2 ounces protein (ricotta and egg whites), 1 simple carbohydrate (jam), and 1 added fat.

Nutritional Profile per Serving
25 g carbohydrate; 12 g protein; 7 g fat;
29% calories from fat; 3 mg cholesterol;
97.5 mg sodium; 211 calories

20

WONDERFUL LUNCHES

Don't skip lunch, don't hit the vending machines, and don't get into a rut! From this point on, lunch can have a different meaning. It doesn't have to be a production, and it doesn't have to take time. However, a healthy lunch does require a little forethought and planning.

Tips for New Lunchtime Fare

‣ *Sandwiches can be a perfect lunch package.*

They give you a perfect balance of complex carbohydrate and protein, and with the right filling they are low-fat as well. Look at the lunch recipes for new sandwich ideas beyond bologna.

If you don't have time to make a fresh sandwich daily, make a week's supply at one time and freeze them. The sandwich will be thawed by lunch, ready to be stuffed with lettuce and other vegetables. Mustard freezes well; mayonnaise does not. Ask your butcher to slice your deli meat so that each slice will give you approximately one ounce. Proper-weight slice will allow for quick and accurate portioning.

‣ *Fast food doesn't have to be a nutritional evil.*

You do have to be responsible, however, for ordering the healthier choices. See chapter seventeen—"Healthy Expectations for Dining Out"—for learning survival in the fast-food lane.

• *If the right food isn't available, in a tight time squeeze you will be apt to reach for the wrong food!*

Have easily stored food items available (such as low-fat cheeses, whole-grain crackers, dried fruits, or Trail Mix) that can be substituted for vending machine fare. A cooler and a thermos can also do wonders for expanding your lunchtime choices.

• *Life in a rut is NO FUN!*

It is easy to have the same hamburger or turkey sandwich every day, but some variety adds a lot in terms of both excitement and nutrition. In winter you might fill an insulated container with a hearty soup or stew. On hot days pack a cold main dish salad in an insulated container. Be sure to review the pages ahead for great ideas of lunches that are perfectly balanced and perfectly delicious!

Packing Safety Pointers

• Keep all food clean. Keep cold foods cold and hot foods hot.

• Your hands, countertops, utensils, and cutting boards should be washed in hot soapy water and rinsed before and after each food preparation time. A thermos, any plastic containers, and the lunch box should be washed and rinsed after each use.

• Bacteria thrives at temperatures between 60 and 125 degrees; food must not be allowed to sit at that temperature for any period of time. Cold foods should be kept at temperatures below 60 degrees maximum and ideally below 40 degrees. Hot foods should be maintained at a temperature above 125 degrees minimum and ideally above 140 degrees. Insulated thermal containers will aid in the fight against room temperatures as they are designed to keep hot foods hot and cold foods cold. Many are designed to double as a bowl and a carrier. What a thermos will *not* do is make cold foods colder or hot foods hotter. Therefore you must give it a good head start. If a cold food or beverage is going into the container, chill it first with ice water or a short stay in the freezer. If hot food is going into the thermos, the container should be preheated with boiling water, and food should be boiling hot when added to maintain desired hot temperatures.

- Sandwiches may be made several days in advance by freezing them. Put a sandwich into the lunch box frozen and allow it to thaw naturally by lunchtime. Cooked meats and poultry freeze very well. Add vegetables to the lunch box to stack on the sandwich before serving. Mayonnaise tends to make the bread soggy when frozen (as well as adding unneeded fat)—avoid it! Mustard is a fine addition and will not make the bread soggy when frozen.

- Freeze your beverage in a plastic container; it will serve as a cold pack to help keep your foods cool. Many lunch boxes also come as minicoolers—made of Styrofoam and containing their own freezer packs.

- Be careful with lunches. With a little help from wise packing, there is brown-bag safety beyond peanut butter sandwiches!

THE LUNCHBOX PACKAGE

WRAPPING	CONTENTS	TRIMMINGS
• whole-wheat, rye, or pumpernickel bread • whole-grain kaiser or hamburger buns • whole-wheat English muffins • low-fat flour tortilla (preferably whole-wheat) • whole-wheat bagels • whole-wheat pita bread • crepes • lettuce leaves • focaccia bread	• lean, sliced meats (turkey, chicken breast, roast beef, Canadian bacon, low-fat ham) • nonfat or low-fat cheese • bean spreads • tuna or salmon • boiled egg whites or tofu • peanut butter and fruit • cottage cheese with Trail Mix	• romaine or leaf lettuce • sliced vegetables (peppers, tomato, cucumbers) • spice sprouts • shredded carrots • mustard or light mayonnaise • salsa

For a lunch that will refresh you, provide for baby, and keep your energy and concentration high, try one of these delicious and fast complete meals.

Pita Pizzas

1 whole-wheat pita, cut in half into rounds (like a saucer)
2 Tbsp. spaghetti sauce
3 oz. or $^3/_4$ cup part-skim or nonfat mozzarella cheese, shredded
1 small apple, cut into wedges

Preheat oven to 375 degrees. Place the two pita circles on a baking sheet. Spread each one with half of the spaghetti sauce and top each with half of the cheese. Bake for 8 to 10 minutes or until cheese is bubbly. Serve with apple wedges.

Makes 1 serving, giving 2 complex carbohydrates (pita bread), 2 ounces protein (cheese), and 1 simple carbohydrate (sauce).

Nutritional profile per serving:
37 g carbohydrate; 22 g protein; 12 g fat;
36% calories from fat; 24 mg cholesterol;
570 mg sodium; 344 calories

Carrot-Cheese Melt

1 grated carrot (about $^1/_2$ cup)
2 oz. grated mozzarella cheese (about $^1/_2$ cup)
2 slices whole-wheat bread
8 oz. skim milk

Mix together carrots and cheese. Spread bread with carrot-cheese mix. Grill in nonstick skillet till cheese melts. Add tomato slices and lettuce (and even alfalfa sprouts).

Makes 1 serving, giving 1 complex carbohydrate (bread), 1 protein (cheese and milk), and 1 simple carbohydrate (carrots).

Nutritional profile per serving:
45 g carbohydrate; 25 g protein; 9 g fat;
22% calories from fat; 24 mg cholesterol;
578 mg sodium; 361 calories

Swiss Stuffed Potatoes

4 baking potatoes (about 5 oz. each)
$^1/_2$ cup part-skim or nonfat ricotta cheese
$^1/_4$ teaspoon salt
$^1/_4$ teaspoon black pepper
6 oz. part-skim or $1^1/_2$ cups nonfat mozzarella cheese, shredded
paprika
2 cups mixed, chopped seasonal fruit

Preheat oven to 400 degrees. Wash the potatoes and bake for 1 hour until done. Or microwave potatoes by pricking and cooking on high for 8 minutes, turning and microwaving for another 8 minutes.

Once cooked, cut the potatoes in half lengthwise and scoop out most of the pulp, leaving a $^1/_4$-inch shell. In a bowl, mash the potato pulp with the ricotta cheese, salt, and pepper. Stir in the mozzarella cheese and spoon the mixture into the potato shells. Sprinkle with paprika.

Increase the oven temperature to broil; broil the stuffed potato shells for 3 to 5 minutes or until they are heated through and lightly browned on top. Serve each potato with $^1/_2$ cup mixed, chopped fruit.

Makes 4 servings of 2 halves each. Each serving gives 1 complex carbohydrate (potato), 2 ounces protein (cheese), and 1 simple carbohydrate (fruit).

Nutritional profile per serving:
28 g carbohydrate; 17 g protein; 9 g fat;
24% calories from fat; 34 mg cholesterol;
513 mg sodium; 339 calories

Turkey Tortilla Roll

1 10-inch whole-wheat flour tortilla
1 tsp. Dijon-style mustard
2 oz. skinned turkey breast, fully cooked and sliced
$^1/_2$ oz. (1 Tbsp.) part-skim milk cheddar cheese, grated
$^1/_2$ tomato, cut into strips
$^1/_4$ cup romaine lettuce, shredded
freshly ground black pepper, if desired
celery and carrot sticks
10 fresh strawberries or other fruit

Spread the tortilla with mustard. Top with the sliced turkey, cheese, tomato, lettuce, and pepper, if desired. Fold in the sides of the tortilla, roll it up burrito-style, and cut it in half. Serve with celery, carrot sticks, and fresh fruit.

Makes 1 serving, giving 1 complex carbohydrate (tortilla), 3 ounces protein (turkey and cheese), and 1 simple carbohydrate (fruit).

Nutritional profile per serving:
31 g carbohydrate; 25 g protein; 7.9 g fat;
24% calories from fat; 49 mg cholesterol;
194 mg sodium; 296 calories

Veggie Sandwich

1 whole-wheat pita
3 oz. cheese (mozzarella, skimmed cheddar, or Alpine Lace "Lean and Free")
a few mushrooms and green pepper rings
sliced tomato

Stuff halved pita with 1 ounce each cheese and vegetables. Microwave on high for 2–3 minutes. Add a couple of tomato slices and be ready for a treat. Serve with a fruit juice spritzer ($^1/_2$ cup juice mixed with club soda or seltzer) over ice.

Makes 1 serving, giving 2 complex carbohydrates (pita), 3 ounces protein (cheese), and simple carbohydrate (juice).

Nutritional profile per serving:
31 g carbohydrate; 25 g protein; 1 g fat;
4% calories from fat; 32 mg cholesterol;
712 mg sodium; 233 calories

Terrific Tuna Grill

2 cans (6^1/2 oz. each) solid white tuna, water-packed, drained
^{1}/2 cup carrots, shredded
1 stalk celery, diced
1 apple, diced (^{1}/2 cup)
2 Tbsp. light mayonnaise
2 Tbsp. orange juice
2 Tbsp. plain, nonfat yogurt
1 tsp. Dijon-style mustard
^{1}/2 tsp. creole seasoning
2 plum tomatoes, sliced
8 slices 100% whole-wheat bread
nonstick cooking spray

Combine the tuna, carrots, celery, and apple. In a separate bowl stir together the mayonnaise, orange juice, yogurt, mustard, and creole seasoning until blended. Pour the mixture over the salad, stirring to coat it. Divide the salad into 4 portions, spreading each portion onto one slice of bread. Top each with 2 slices of tomato and the other slice of bread. Spray a nonstick skillet with nonstick cooking spray and heat on medium high. Grill the sandwiches until brown.

Makes 4 servings, each giving 2 complex carbohydrates (bread), 3 ounces protein (tuna), and 1 simple carbohydrate (veggies and fruit).

Nutritional profile per serving:
37 g carbohydrate; 28 g protein; 4.7 g fat;
14% calories from fat; 38 mg cholesterol;
567 mg sodium; 300 calories

Grilled Turkey and Cheese Sandwich

2 teaspoons Dijon-style mustard
2 slices 100% whole-wheat bread
1 oz. (^{1}/4 cup) Jarlsberg Lite cheese, grated
1 ripe plum tomato, sliced
2 oz. skinned turkey breast, fully cooked and sliced
nonstick cooking spray
1 cup watermelon chunks

Spread the mustard on each slice of bread. Put 2 tablespoons of cheese, the tomato, and the turkey on one slice of bread. Sprinkle with the additional cheese and top with the remaining slice of bread. Grill the sandwich on a hot griddle or a nonstick skillet coated with nonstick spray. Cook until the bread is lightly browned and the cheese melts. Serve with the melon.

Makes 1 serving, giving 2 complex carbohydrates (bread), 3 ounces protein (turkey and cheese), and 1 simple carbohydrate (fruit).

Nutritional profile per serving:
32 g carbohydrate; 29 g protein; 7 g fat;
20.5% calories from fat; 62 mg cholesterol;
551 mg sodium; 307 calories

Chicken of the Land or Sea Apple Sandwich

³/₄ cup water-packed tuna or chicken
1 small stalk of chopped celery
1 Tbsp. reduced-calorie mayonnaise
1 small chopped apple
1 whole-wheat pita
romaine lettuce leaves

Mix together first 4 ingredients. Stuff into 2 halves of pita lined with lettuce.

Makes 1 serving, giving 2 complex carbohydrates (pita), 3 protein (chicken), 1 simple carbohydrate (fruit), and added fat (mayonnaise).

Nutritional profile per serving:
42 g carbohydrate; 25 g protein; 8 g fat;
30% calories from fat; 40 g cholesterol;
650 mg sodium; 233 calories

Chicken and Pasta Salad

12 oz. smoked (or roasted) chicken breast
1 recipe of Greek Pasta*
2 cups fresh spinach, washed, stemmed, and snipped
2 cups romaine or red leaf lettuce
1 cup radicchio leaves, torn or extra romaine
4 plum tomatoes, quartered
$^1/_2$ cup feta cheese, crumbled
$^1/_4$ cup Greek Vinaigrette**
2 Tbsp. chopped fresh herbs (cilantro, basil, rosemary, thyme)

Cut chicken breast into chunks; mix with Greek Pasta. Place spinach, romaine, and radicchio on each of four plates; top with pasta salad. Add tomatoes and crumbled feta cheese. Ladle 1 tablespoon of Greek Vinaigrette onto each plate, then sprinkle with herbs.

Serves 4, each giving 2 complex carbohydrates (pasta, spinach, lettuce, and radicchio), 4 ounces of protein (chicken and cheese), and 1 simple carbohydrate.

Nutritional profile per serving:
28 g protein; 41 g carbohydrate; 9 g fat;
22% calories from fat; 0 mg cholesterol;
720 mg sodium; 357 calories

*Greek Pasta

4 cups bowtie pasta, cooked and cooled
1 red bell pepper, finely diced
1 green bell pepper, finely diced
1 yellow pepper, finely diced
$^1/_2$ red onion, finely minced
2 Tbsp. chopped fresh herbs (cilantro, basil, rosemary, thyme)
1 cup Greek Vinaigrette (recipe follows)
1 tsp. creole seasoning

Combine all ingredients. Allow to marinate at least one hour.
Makes 4 servings. Each serving gives 2 complex carbohydrates (pasta) and 1 ounce protein.

Nutritional profile per serving:
7 g protein; 35 g carbohydrate; 4 g fat;
18% calories from fat; 0 mg cholesterol;
420 mg sodium; 204 calories

**Greek Vinaigrette

$^1/_4$ cup olive oil
$1^1/_4$ cups rice wine vinegar
$^3/_4$ cup chicken stock (fat-free/low salt)
$^1/_4$ cup Dijon mustard
$^1/_2$ cup pepperoncini juice
1 Tbsp. minced garlic
1 Tbsp. minced shallots
1 tsp. creole seasoning
2 Tbsp. chopped fresh herbs (cilantro, basil, rosemary, thyme)
1 Tbsp. chopped fresh oregano (or 1 tsp. dried)

In a large bowl, whisk together ingredients. Refrigerate. Makes 24 servings, 2 tablespoons each.

Nutritional profile per serving:
0 g protein; 1 g carbohydrate; 2 g fat;
66% calories from fat; 0 mg cholesterol;
139 mg sodium; 21 calories

Quick Mexican Chili

1 lb. ground turkey
1 small onion, diced
1 small green pepper
1 can (15^1/2 oz.) tomato sauce
1 can (15^1/2 oz.) crushed tomatoes
1 can (15^1/2 oz.) kidney beans, rinsed
2 tsp. chili powder
1 tsp. garlic powder
^{1}/2 tsp. creole seasoning
1^1/2 cups brown rice, cooked

Crumble the ground turkey into a hard plastic colander. Microwave the turkey on high for 3 minutes; stir and break it apart. Add the onion and the green pepper. Microwave another 3 to 4 minutes until the turkey is browned. Spoon the meat and the vegetables into a saucepan and add the remaining ingredients. Cook the mixture over medium-high heat until it boils. Simmer uncovered for 10 more minutes, stirring to prevent it from burning.

Serve over ^{1}/4 cup cooked brown rice in a large soup bowl. Freeze the remaining servings in individual freezer bags for later use.

Makes 6 servings (1^1/2 cups each), giving 1 complex carbohydrate (rice), 3 ounces protein (turkey and beans), and 1 simple carbohydrate (veggies).

Nutritional profile per serving:
32 g carbohydrate; 25 g protein; 1 g fat;
4% calories from fat; 47 mg cholesterol;
742 mg sodium; 237 calories

Smoked Turkey and White Bean Soup

1 tsp. olive oil
2 cloves garlic, minced
1 can (14 oz.) whole tomatoes, drained
2 Tbsp. chopped fresh basil (or 2 tsp. dried)
6 cups chicken stock (fat-free/low salt)
2 cans (19 oz. each) or 4 cups cooked
    cannelini or white beans, drained and rinsed
1 lb. smoked turkey, rough chopped
$^1/_2$ tsp. creole seasoning
1 tsp. Mrs. Dash seasoning

Spray a large stockpot with cooking spray. Add olive oil and bring to low heat. Add garlic and cook, stirring, about 1 minute. Add tomatoes and basil; simmer for 5 minutes, crushing the tomatoes with stirring spoon. Pour in chicken stock and simmer over medium heat.

Stir in cannelini beans and smoked turkey along with the seasonings. Heat through. Serve with mixed green salad.

Makes 5 servings (3 cups each), giving 2 complex carbohydrates (beans), 4 ounces protein (turkey and beans), 1 simple carbohydrate (tomatoes), and added fat (olive oil).

Nutritional profile per serving:
38 g protein; 34 g carbohydrates; 8 g fat;
20% calories from fat; 66 mg cholesterol;
1120 mg sodium; 364 calories

Vegetable Tortilla Pizza

2 fajita-sized, fat-free flour tortillas
$^2/_3$ cup fat-free mozzarella/Parmesan cheese blend, divided
   (2 parts mozzarella, 1 part Parmesan)
$^1/_4$ cup Classico Tomato & Basil Sauce
1 Tbsp. chopped fresh herbs (cilantro, basil, rosemary,
   thyme), divided
6 strips red bell pepper
6 strips green bell pepper
6 strips yellow bell pepper
3 broccoli florets
$^1/_4$ small red onion, diced

Preheat oven to 450 degrees.

Lay one tortilla on round wire mesh pan. Sprinkle it with 2 tablespoons cheese blend; top with remaining tortilla.

Brush the top of tortilla with Tomato & Basil Sauce and sprinkle with $^1/_2$ tablespoon herbs. Lay peppers, broccoli, and onions on top of sauce. Sprinkle with the remaining cheese blend.

Bake until lightly browned and crisp, about 5 minutes. Sprinkle with remaining herbs.

Makes 1 serving, giving 2 complex carbohydrates (tortillas), 4 ounces of protein (cheese blend), 1 simple carbohydrate (tomato sauce).

Nutritional profile per serving:
36 g protein; 48 g carbohydrate; 10 g fat;
21% calories from fat; 64 mg cholesterol;
700 mg sodium; 426 calories

21

EASY, DELICIOUS, AND
HEALTHY DINNERS

There are times when having a basic format from which to work can be invaluable! These are meals that you can use as a beginning place: They are perfectly balanced, everyone will like them, and they are easy!

Cooking-Quick Survival Tips

- Keep your pantry, fridge, and freezer well-stocked with the basic ingredients for quick and easy food preparation.

- Keep an ongoing grocery list and jot down items as soon as you begin to run low. If you wait until you are completely out of an item, it could cost you an unplanned trip to the store.

- After you have shopped, plan to use the most perishable foods first: fresh seafood, leafy vegetables, and some fruits. Saving the hardiest foods for last will help reduce waste and eliminate unnecessary trips to the store.

- Since half the battle is just deciding what to prepare, pick out the meal you are going to try one or two days in advance—and make sure you have the needed ingredients on hand. If you have a family, enlist them in this time of preparing—even allow them the responsibility for a meal or two each week.

- A recipe generally takes longer the first time you prepare it, so when you plan to make a new dish give yourself the extra edge of time.

- These dishes are designed for your time and effort to be spent on one part of the meal. If the entrée requires a bit more time to prepare, it is put together with a simpler side dish.

- Keep a ready-to-cook kitchen: Do most of your food preparation on a countertop close to your sink. Declutter your countertops by storing your seldom used appliances in less accessible cabinets. Use the drawer and cabinet closest to your cooking area to store knives, vegetable scrub brushes and peelers, stirring spoons, measuring spoons and cups, mixing bowls, colanders, cutting boards, scales, and graters. Keep your food processor and hand-held blender close so they are always handy for quick chopping, mincing, or blending.

Freeze properly portioned leftovers in Ziploc freezer bags for quick meals when you need them most!

Trimming Time by Freezing Food

A major part of living the good life is not to spend any unnecessary time in the kitchen! My theory about cooking is, and has always been, "If it takes longer to cook it than to eat it, FORGET IT!" How about you?

One way to streamline your food preparation is to look for the recipes that can be doubled or tripled, then frozen for later use. Nothing can calm frenzied nerves after a busy day—overflowing into a busy night—like a meal that can be pulled out and heated up in a jiffy!

If you're marinating and grilling two chicken breasts, why not do a dozen? Then you can freeze them individually in small plastic zip-top bags. Later they can be popped into the microwave for a quick chicken sandwich or salad. The same goes for any number of dishes —from lasagna to meatloaf.

I also use this theory when I'm picking up takeout. Rather then getting two Chinese meals to bring home, I bring home four and freeze the two extras in small bags for quick meals. Combined with my own flavorful brown rice, it makes a terrific treat days later.

And don't forget about freezing some of the use-in-everything ingredients like stocks, sauces, and chopped veggies. They can be frozen in small quantities perfectly sized for your recipes.

Tips for Fantasic Freezing

- Keep your eyes and mind open for doubling up on recipes, saving you time and effort later. Highlight those recipes to remind you even before you go to the store.

- Choose foods to freeze wisely: Some foods just don't freeze well. The higher the fat content, the shorter its storage potential. And foods that are high in water content will turn to mush, like tomatoes, lettuces, and other salad vegetables. Milk and yogurt sauces will curdle.

- Cool food quickly before you freeze it. Don't let your flavor-packed, texture-filled food sit around and lose its quality. Put it in the freezing container, seal it, then cool it in very cold water before freezing.

- Pack it small and flat, using quart-size, heavy-duty, sealable plastic freezer bags. Pack in individual portion sizes so that you can prepare for one, two, or four. Fill bags with food, press out the air, seal, and freeze so they are flat. I place them in boxes according to proteins, complex carbohydrates, and simple carbohydrate vegetables. Just a simple shoebox will do.

- Date each bag. And name it, too! I jot down names and dates with a permanent ink pen. Use your frozen foods within six months.

- Defrost carefully. Don't ever leave food out at room temperature for over three hours to thaw. Thaw overnight in the refrigerator or microwave them on defrost (30 percent power) for six to eight minutes per pound of food.

- Combine a frozen meal with a fresh food. This will give you a great balance of aroma, nutrients, color, and texture.

After a month of cooking for your immediate meal plus making extra to store in the freezer, it won't be necessary to cook but two or three times a week—because there is always something special waiting for you in that special place!

1

Hawaiian Chicken (3 ounces protein)
Wild Rice Pilaf (1 complex carbohydrate)
Sliced Tomatoes (healthy munchie)
Green Beans and Mushrooms (1 simple carbohydrate)

Hawaiian Chicken

$^1/_3$ cup unsweetened pineapple juice
$^1/_3$ cup low-sodium soy sauce
$^1/_3$ cup sherry or alcohol-free Chardonnay
4 skinned chicken breasts
2 cloves garlic
1 Tbsp. parsley
ground pepper to taste

Mix all but chicken. Marinate chicken breasts (skinned, deboned, and split lengthwise) for 3–4 hours or overnight. (The marinade adds no significant calories.) Grill. Makes 4 servings.

Nutritional profile per serving:
5 g carbohydrate; 27 g protein; 3 g fat;
16% calories from fat; 72 g cholesterol;
126 mg sodium; 182 calories

Wild Rice Pilaf

1 tsp. olive oil
1 medium onion, chopped
1 clove minced garlic
1 stalk celery, chopped
2 cups chicken broth
$^1/_4$ cup wild rice
$^3/_4$ cup brown rice
$^1/_4$ tsp. salt (optional)
1 Tbsp. parsley

Sauté vegetables in medium saucepan with 1 teaspoon olive oil. Add broth and optional salt; bring to boil and add rices. Boil for one minute;

reduce heat and simmer for 45 mintues until the liquid is absorbed. Garnish with parsley. Makes 6 $^1\!/_2$-cup servings.

Nutritional profile per serving:
21 g carbohydrate; 4 g protein; 2 g fat;
22% calories from fat; 0 mg cholesterol;
210 mg sodium; 122 calories

Green Beans and Mushrooms

1 tsp. olive oil
1 clove minced garlic
$^1\!/_2$ lb. washed mushrooms
$^1\!/_2$ tsp. rosemary
$^1\!/_2$ tsp. basil
1 Tbsp. parsley
$^1\!/_2$ tsp. salt (optional)
$^1\!/_4$ tsp. pepper
1 lb. steamed green beans

Sauté olive oil, garlic, and mushrooms in nonstick pan for 3–4 minutes. Add spices and simmer covered for 1 more minute. Toss well with beans. Makes 4 servings.

Nutritional profile per serving:
9 g carbohydrate; 2 g protein; 2 g fat;
17% calories from fat; 0 mg cholesterol;
4 mg sodium; 129 calories

2 Sicilian Chicken and Pasta (3 ounces protein, 1 complex carbohydrate, and 1 simple carbohydrate) Marinated Cucumbers (your healthy munchie)

Sicilian Chicken and Pasta

4 boneless, skinless chicken breasts
$1/2$ tsp. creole seasoning
$1/2$ tsp. dried basil
$1/2$ tsp. dried oregano
2 cans ($15^1/2$ oz.) Italian-style stewed tomatoes
2 Tbsp. cornstarch
$1/4$ tsp. Tabasco sauce
1 clove minced garlic
$1/4$ cup grated Parmesan cheese
1 small package of angel hair pasta (8 oz.)

Preheat the oven to 425 degrees. Sprinkle the chicken with the seasoning and pat it with the herbs. Place the chicken in a baking dish and cover it with foil. Bake for 15 minutes.

While the chicken is baking, pour the canned tomatoes into a medium saucepan and add the cornstarch, the Tabasco sauce, and the garlic. Cook the mixture until it is thickened, about 5 minutes.

After 15 minutes, remove the chicken from the oven, pouring off any liquid from the pan. Pour the heated sauce over the chicken and sprinkle the grated cheese on top. Place the pan back in the oven and cook, uncovered, for 10 more minutes. Cook the pasta according to the package directions. Drain and place it on a platter. Top the pasta with the chicken and the sauce.

Makes 4 servings.

Nutritional profile per serving:
27 g carbohydrate; 25 g protein; 9 g fat;
20% calories from fat; 50 mg cholesterol;
878 mg sodium; 396 calories

Marinated Cucumbers

4 cucumbers
1 small red onion, thinly sliced
1 tsp. dried dill weed
$1/2$ cup no-oil Italian dressing
4 romaine or green leaf lettuce leaves

Wash and peel the cucumbers; slice in rounds. Add the onion slices and toss with the dill weed. Pour in the dressing and refrigerate at least 2 hours to blend the flavors. Serve on a lettuce leaf.

Makes 8 servings of a healthy munchie.

Nutritional profile per serving:
9 g carbohydrate; 1 g protein; 0 g fat;
0% calories from fat; 0 mg cholesterol;
280 mg sodium; 40 calories

3

Shrimp Creole (3 ounces protein and
1 complex carbohydrate)
Steamed Broccoli (2 simple carbohydrates)
Caesar Salad (your healthy munchie and an added fat)

Shrimp Creole

White Wine Worcestershire sauce
1 lb. fresh medium shrimp
nonstick cooking spray
2 tsp. olive oil
2 cloves garlic, finely chopped
1 small red onion, finely chopped
$^1/_2$ teaspoon creole seasoning
2 cups tomato purée, canned
$^1/_2$ cup chicken stock, defatted
2 plum tomatoes, cut lengthwise into strips
2 cups brown rice, cooked
1 lemon wedge
sprinkle of fresh chopped herbs (such as basil or thyme)
2 cups broccoli, steamed

Marinate the shrimp in Worcestershire sauce for 1 hour. Spray nonstick skillet with nonstick cooking spray; heat with 2 teaspoons of olive oil. Add garlic and onions and sauté until they are softened and transparent. Season shrimp with creole seasoning and sauté quickly in the hot pan.

Add tomato purée and chicken stock, heating through. Add tomato strips at the end of cooking.

Mound $^1/_2$ cup rice in the center of each of four plates; spoon $^1/_4$ of shrimp and sauce over each rice mound. Garnish with a lemon wedge and sprinkle with the chopped herbs. Serve with the steamed broccoli.

Makes 4 servings.

Nutritional profile per serving:
38 g carbohydrate; 23 g protein; 4 g fat;
14% calories from fat; 66 mg cholesterol;
357 mg sodium; 279 calories

Caesar Salad

4 cups romaine lettuce, washed and torn
1 clove minced garlic
$1^1/_2$ Tbsp. olive oil
$^1/_2$ tsp. dry mustard
1 tsp. Worcestershire sauce
$^1/_8$ tsp. coarse black pepper
$^1/_8$ tsp. salt (optional)
1 coddled egg*
juice of 1 lemon
$^1/_4$ cup Parmesan cheese, grated
croutons (from 2 slices whole-wheat bread sprinkled with garlic
  powder and toasted until brown)

Rub the bottom and sides of a large salad bowl with the garlic; leave the garlic in the bowl. Add the oil, the mustard, the Worcestershire sauce, and the spices; beat together with a fork or wire whisk. Add the chilled romaine lettuce; toss well. Crack the coddled egg over the salad; add the lemon juice and toss until the lettuce is well covered. Top with the Parmesan cheese and croutons. Toss well and enjoy!

Makes 6 servings.

*Coddle an egg by immersing the egg in its shell in boiling water for 30 seconds. This makes it safe to eat.

Nutritional profile per serving:
6 g carbohydrate; 4 g protein; 5 g fat;
51% calories from fat; 39 mg cholesterol;
152 mg sodium; 81 calories

4

Black Bean Soup Over Rice (2 ounces protein
and 2 complex carbohydrates)
Spinach and Apple Salad (1 simple carbohydrate)

Black Bean Soup Over Rice

nonstick cooking spray
2 tsp. olive oil
2 cloves garlic, finely chopped
1 small red onion, diced
2 cups chicken stock, defatted
4 cups cooked black beans (if canned, rinse and drain)
1 tsp. creole seasoning
1 tsp. ground cumin
2 cups brown rice, cooked
3 limes, halved
1 cilantro leaf (optional)

Spray a nonstick pan with nonstick cooking spray. Heat the olive oil in the pan. Add the onion and the garlic; sauté until translucent. Add the chicken stock, $2^{1}/2$ cups of the cooked black beans, and the creole seasoning. Bring the mixture to a gentle boil and cook until the amount is reduced by a third; purée in a blender or food processor until smooth. (You may refrigerate this now for serving later. Then reheat the bean purée; if necessary, thin the purée with additional chicken stock to make it smooth.)

When serving, place cup of the cooked brown rice in each of 6 bowls. Top with $^{1}/4$ cup of the reserved whole black beans. Add 1 cup heated bean purée. Squeeze $^{1}/2$ lime over each bowl. Garnish with a cilantro leaf if desired.

Makes 6 servings.

Nutritional profile per serving:
47 g carbohydrate; 12 g protein; 3 g fat;
12% calories from fat; 0 mg cholesterol;
367 mg sodium; 261 calories

Spinach and Apple Salad

2 Tbsp. canola oil
$1^{1}/_{2}$ tsp. basil
1 tsp. onion powder
$^{1}/_{2}$ tsp. salt (optional)
$^{1}/_{8}$ tsp. pepper
$^{3}/_{4}$ cup apple juice
2 Tbsp. apple cider vinegar
$^{1}/_{2}$ cup orange segments
4 cups spinach, torn in pieces
2 cups apple, thinly sliced

In a small bowl prepare the dressing by combining the oil, basil, onion powder, salt, and pepper; set aside for 10 minutes to allow the flavors to blend. Stir in the apple juice and vinegar. In a large bowl, combine the spinach, apple, and oranges. Toss with $^{1}/_{2}$ cup dressing; serve immediately. Refrigerate the remaining dressing for other salads or a marinade.

Makes 6 servings.

Nutritional profile per serving:
12 g carbohydrate; 1 g protein; 2 g fat;
26% calories from fat; 0 mg cholesterol;
30 mg sodium; 69 calories

5

Dijon-Crusted Salmon (3 ounces protein)
Baked Sweet Potato (1 complex carbohydrate)
Tuscan Broccoli (1 simple carbohydrate)

Dijon-Crusted Salmon

4 salmon fillets, 5 oz. each
White Wine Worcestershire sauce to cover fish
nonstick cooking spray
1 tsp. olive oil
$1/2$ tsp. creole seasoning
4 Tbsp. Dijon-style mustard
4 Tbsp. toasted bread crumbs
2 Tbsp. chopped fresh parsley

Marinate the fish in White Wine Worcestershire sauce for at least 15 minutes to 1 hour. Preheat oven to 350 degrees. Spray a nonstick skillet with nonstick cooking spray and heat it with the olive oil. Sprinkle the marinated fish with creole seasoning and sear it quickly in the hot pan. Spread the top of each fillet with 1 tablespoon mustard; then sprinkle on 1 tablespoon bread crumbs and $1/2$ tablespoon chopped parsley. Place the fillets in the hot oven and roast until they are browned and done, approximately 8 to 10 minutes.

Makes 4 servings.

Nutritional profile per serving:
6 g carbohydrate; 25 g protein; 8.8 g fat;
39% calories from fat; 42 mg cholesterol;
434 mg sodium; 207 calories

Baked Sweet Potatoes

2 medium sweet potatoes
cinnamon (optional)

Preheat oven to 400 degrees. Wash and scrub 2 sweet potatoes. Place them on the oven rack, baking for 45 minutes or until fork tender. Or prick the scrubbed sweet potatoes with a fork and microwave on high for 4 minutes. Turn the sweet potatoes over and microwave another 4 minutes.

When serving, cut the potatoes in half and fluff with a fork; sprinkle with cinnamon, if desired.

Makes 4 servings.

Nutritional profile per serving:
14 g carbohydrate; 1 g protein; 0 g fat;
0% calories from fat; 0 mg cholesterol;
6 mg sodium; 60 calories

Tuscan Broccoli

1 tsp. olive oil
2 cloves garlic, minced
2 Tbsp. capers, rinsed
$^1\!/_2$ tsp. creole seasoning
1 tsp. Mrs. Dash seasoning
1 Tbsp. chopped fresh rosemary (or 1 tsp. dried)
$^1\!/_2$ cup chicken stock (fat-free/low salt)
1 bunch (1$^1\!/_4$ lbs.) broccoli, cut into florets and trimmed of tough stalks

Spray a large nonstick skillet with cooking spray. Add olive oil and heat over medium heat. Add garlic, capers, seasonings, and rosemary; sauté until the garlic is golden, about 30 seconds. Add the broccoli florets and chicken stock. Reduce heat and cook covered until broccoli is crisp tender and cooking liquid is reduced, about 5 to 7 minutes. Ladle into serving dish, tossing together.

Makes 4 servings.

Nutritional profile per serving:
8 g carbohydrate; 4 g protein; 1 g fat;
16% calories from fat; 0 mg cholesterol;
688 mg sodium; 57 calories

6

Snapper With Tomato and Feta Cheese
(4 ounces protein and $^{1}/_{2}$ simple carbohydrate)
Corn on the Cob (1 complex carbohydrate)
Cabbage Slaw (your healthy munchie and
$^{1}/_{2}$ simple carbohydrate)

Snapper With Tomato and Feta Cheese

2 ripe tomatoes, sliced
2 cloves garlic, finely minced
1 lb. red snapper fillets ($^{1}/_{2}$-inch thick)
1 tsp. dried basil
1 lemon, thinly sliced
$^{1}/_{2}$ tsp. dried oregano
$^{1}/_{3}$ cup feta cheese, crumbled

Arrange the tomato slices on the bottom of a 9-inch glass pie dish. Sprinkle the garlic over the tomatoes and arrange the fish over the top. Sprinkle the basil over the fish.

Place the lemon slices on top; sprinkle with the oregano and the crumbled feta cheese. If possible, let the fish sit for about 30 minutes.

Cover the fish with vented plastic wrap and microwave on high for $4^{1}/_{2}$ to 5 minutes. Let it stand for 5 minutes.

Makes 4 servings.

Nutritional profile per serving:
7 g carbohydrate; 27 g protein; 6 g fat;
28% calories from fat; 60 mg cholesterol;
318 mg sodium; 190 calories

Cabbage Slaw

3 cups shredded cabbage
1 cup shredded red cabbage
1 cup shredded carrot
$^{1}/_{4}$ cup finely chopped onion
$^{1}/_{4}$ cup rice wine vinegar
$^{1}/_{4}$ cup unsweetened pineapple juice
1 Tbsp. Dijon-style mustard
$^{1}/_{8}$ tsp. salt
$^{1}/_{8}$ tsp. pepper

Combine the cabbages, carrot, and onion in a medium bowl; toss gently.
Combine the vinegar with the remaining ingredients and stir well. Add to
the cabbage mixture and toss gently. Cover and chill at least 1 hour.

Makes 8 servings ($^{1}/_{2}$ cup each).

Nutritional profile per serving:
5 g carbohydrate; 1 g protein; 2 g fat;
43% calories from fat; 0 mg cholesterol;
124 mg sodium; 42 calories

7

Marvelous Meat Loaf (3 ounces protein and
   1 complex carbohydrate)
Corn on the Cob (1 complex carbohydrate)
Colorful Green Beans (1 simple carbohydrate)
Romaine Salad (your healthy munchie)

Marvelous Meat Loaf

2 lbs. ground round or ground turkey
2 cups old-fashioned oats
$3/4$ cup minced onion
$1/4$ green pepper, minced
2 eggs, slightly beaten
$1/2$ tsp. salt
$1/2$ tsp. pepper
1 Tbsp. Worcestershire sauce
1 tsp. dry mustard
$1/4$ cup skim milk
$3/4$ cup tomato sauce

In large bowl, mix together all ingredients except $1/2$ cup of the tomato sauce. Shape meat into 2 loaves and place in loaf pans sprayed with cooking spray. Spread the additional $1/2$ cup tomato sauce on top. Bake in 400 degree oven for 40 minutes. Makes 10 servings.

Nutritional profile per serving:
11 g carbohydrate; 22 g protein; 9 g fat;
25% calories from fat; 98 mg cholesterol;
257 mg sodium; 213 calories

Colorful Green Beans

1 lb. green beans
$^1/_2$ cup chopped onion
$^1/_2$ tsp. salt (optional)
$^1/_4$ tsp. pepper
2 medium tomatoes, peeled and cut into 8 wedges
1 tsp. olive oil
$^1/_2$ cup chopped celery

Remove strings from beans; wash and cut diagonally into 2-inch pieces. Heat oil in skillet, add onion and celery to skillet, and sauté until tender; add beans, salt, and pepper. Cover and simmer 10 minutes, stirring occasionally. Add tomato; cover and cook an additional 5 minutes. Makes 4 servings.

Nutritional profile per serving:
9 g carbohydrate; 2 g protein; 1 g fat;
17% calories from fat; 0 mg cholesterol;
4 mg sodium; 53 calories

8

Turkey Burgers (4 ounces protein and
 2 complex carbohydrates)
Raw Veggies With Yogurt Dip (your healthy munchie)
Watermelon Quarters (1 simple carbohydrate)

Turkey Burgers

3 lb. ground turkey breast
8 oz. refrigerated hash browns or shredded raw potato
$1/4$ cup chopped parsley
1 Tbsp. creole seasoning
2 Tbsp. tablespoons minced garlic
$1/3$ cup diced white onions
4 oz. chicken stock, defatted
2 egg whites or $1/4$ cup egg substitute
whole-wheat hamburger buns

Crumble the turkey into a bowl. Spray a nonstick pan with nonstick cooking spray; heat. Add the shredded hash browns and brown. Let the hash browns cool and then add them to the turkey with the remaining ingredients. Shape into 10 patties. Grill the patties and serve on whole-wheat hamburger buns. The remaining patties may be frozen individually in freezer bags, before or after cooking. If the patties are frozen uncooked, thaw them in the refrigerator before grilling.
Makes 10 servings.

Nutritional profile per serving:
36 g carbohydrate; 30 g protein; 6.5 g fat;
19% calories from fat; 96 mg cholesterol;
244 mg sodium; 330 calories

Raw Veggies With Yogurt Dip

1 cup skim milk
$1/2$ cup nonfat plain yogurt
2 Tbsp. dried minced onion
2 Tbsp. lemon juice
$1/2$ tsp. garlic powder
$1/2$ tsp. salt (optional)
$1/2$ tsp. dried oregano
1 tsp. dried parsley
$1/2$ tsp. onion powder
$1/4$ tsp. black pepper
raw vegetables

Mix all the ingredients for the dip together and chill. Serve with raw vegetables.

Makes 12 1-ounce servings of 2 tablespoons each.

Nutritional profile per serving:
1 g carbohydrate; 1 g protein; 0 g fat;
0% calories from fat; 0 mg cholesterol;
107 mg sodium; 12 calories

9

Zesty Chicken Quesadillas (4 ounces protein and
2 complex carbohydrates)
Sliced Melon (1 simple carbohydrate)

Zesty Chicken Quesadillas

4 10-inch whole-wheat flour tortillas
4 skinless, boneless chicken breasts or 2 cans (6^{1}/2 oz. each) of
white-meat chicken
1 yellow, red, or green pepper
2 tomatoes, diced
4 oz. part-skim cheddar cheese, grated
2 oz. mixed greens: romaine, red leaf, Bibb
1 cup cooked black beans (if canned, rinse)
^{1}/4 cup picante sauce
cantaloupe, peeled and sliced

Cut the chicken breasts into lengthwise strips and poach or grill until
tender. If using canned chicken, drain the 2 cans of white-meat chicken.
Dice the peppers. Lay the tortilla in a large, heated nonstick skillet. Sprinkle
^{1}/4 of the chicken breast strips, the diced peppers, the diced tomatoes, and
the cheese on one half of each tortilla. Fold over the other half of the tortilla
and grill until it is browned and crispy and the cheese is melted.

Cut each quesadilla into 3 triangles and lay each piece on a plate next to
the greens. Top the greens with the black beans. Serve with picante sauce
for dipping. Lay cantaloupe slices to the side of the plate.

Makes 4 servings.

Nutritional profile per serving:
40 g carbohydrate; 32 g protein; 10 g fat;
23% calories from fat; 66 mg cholesterol;
751 mg sodium; 385 calories

10

Oven-Baked Chicken (3 ounces protein)
Peas Rosemary (1 complex carbohydrate)
Carrot Salad à la Difference
(1 simple carbohydrate)

Oven-Baked Chicken

2 egg whites, lightly beaten
2 cups Nutri-Grain Golden Wheat cereal, crushed
$^1/_4$ tsp. pepper
6 chicken half-breasts, deboned and skinned
1 Tbsp. water
$^1/_4$ tsp. garlic powder
$^1/_4$ tsp. seasoned salt (optional)

Mix together egg and water in shallow dish; set aside. Combine crushed cereal and spices. Dip chicken in egg mixture, then dredge in cereal mixture, coating well. Arrange in baking pan coated with cooking spray. Bake, uncovered, at 350 degrees for 45 minutes, or until tender. It tastes like fried chicken! Yields 6 servings.

Nutritional profile per serving:
7 g carbohydrate; 27 g protein; 4 g fat;
21% calories from fat; 108 mg cholesterol;
123 mg sodium; 176 calories

Carrot Salad à la Difference

1 lb. coarsely grated carrots
2 medium apples, grated
1 cup firm plain, nonfat yogurt
$^1/_2$ cup crushed unsweetened pineapple
$^1/_2$ cup raisins

Combine all ingredients and chill. Makes 12 1-cup servings.

Nutrional profile per serving:
14 g carbohydrate; 2 g protein; 0 g fat;
0% calories from fat; 0 g cholesterol;
28 mg sodium; 62 calories

Peas Rosemary

1 pkg. frozen peas, cooked and drained
2 tsp. olive oil
2 cloves minced garlic
$^1/_4$ cup chopped onion
$^1/_4$ tsp. pepper
1 tsp. rosemary
$^1/_4$ tsp. salt (optional)

Sauté garlic and onion in oil until tender. Add rosemary, salt, and pepper; continue to sauté one more minute. Toss with peas. Makes 4 servings.

Nutritional profile per serving:
12 g carbohydrate; 4 g protein; 2 g fat;
23% calories from fat; 0 mg cholesterol;
95 mg sodium; 83 calories

11

Stir-fry Chicken With Snow Peas (2-3 ounces protein and 1 simple carbohydrate)
Apple Walnut Salad (1 simple carbohydrate)

Stir-Fry Chicken With Snow Peas

2 cloves garlic, minced
2 Tbsp. low-sodium soy sauce
1 Tbsp. sherry
2 Tbsp. cornstarch
2 split chicken breasts, cut into 1-inch cubes
20 snow pea pods, sliced
$1/2$ cup water chestnuts, drained
$1/2$ cup chicken stock
2 tsp. peanut or canola oil

Mix together garlic, soy sauce, sherry, and cornstarch; marinate chicken pieces in mixture for 15 minutes. Spray wok with nonstick cooking spray, then heat with 2 tsp. peanut oil. Add chicken; stir-fry for 30 seconds. Add chicken broth; stir-fry until thickened. Serve immediately. Wonderful over brown rice. Makes 2 servings. The brown rice would be your complex carbohydrate.

Nutritional profile per serving:
15 g carbohydrate; 28 g protein; 7 g fat;
27% calories from fat 72 mg cholesterol;
126 mg sodium; 235 calories

Apple Walnut Salad

2 Granny Smith apples, cored and sliced thin
2 Tbsp. chopped walnuts
2 Tbsp. chicken stock (fat-free/low salt)
1 Tbsp. white wine vinegar
2 tsp. walnut oil (or olive oil)
1 Tbsp. finely chopped shallots
1 tsp. Dijon mustard
$^1/_4$ tsp. salt
$^1/_4$ tsp. cracked black pepper
8 cups washed, dried, and torn mixed greens (red leaf, romaine, frizee, radicchio, arugula, or bibb)

In a small, dry skillet over low heat, stir walnuts until lightly toasted, about 3 minutes. Transfer to a plate to cool.

In a large salad bowl, whisk together chicken stock, vinegar, oil, shallots, mustard, salt, and pepper. Add greens and apples and toss thoroughly. Sprinkle with the toasted walnuts.

Nutritional profile per serving:
14 g carbohydrate; 2.5 g protein; 4 g fat;
35% calories from fat; 0 mg cholesterol;
159 mg sodium; 91 calories

12

Spaghetti Pie (2 ounces protein, 1 complex
carbohydrate, and 1 simple carbohydrate)
Marinated Veggies**
Fresh Fruit Salad

Spaghetti Pie

6 oz. vermicelli or whole-wheat pasta
2 tsp. olive oil
$^1/_3$ cup grated Parmesan cheese
2 egg whites, well beaten
$^1/_2$ lb. ground turkey*
$^1/_2$ cup chopped onion
$^1/_4$ cup chopped green pepper
8 oz. can stewed tomatoes
6 oz. can tomato paste
$^3/_4$ tsp. dried oregano
$^1/_4$ tsp. salt (optional)
$^1/_2$ tsp. garlic powder
1 cup part-skimmed ricotta cheese
$^1/_2$ cup shredded mozzarella cheese

Cook pasta according to package directions; drain. Stir olive oil and
Parmesan cheese into hot pasta. Add egg whites, stirring well. Spoon mixture into a 10-inch pie plate. Use a spoon to shape the spaghetti into a pie
shell. Microwave uncovered on high 3 minutes or until set. Set aside.

Crumble turkey in a colander, stir in onion and green pepper. Cover with
plastic wrap and microwave on high 5–6 minutes, stirring every 2 mintues.
Let drain well. Put into a bowl and stir in tomatoes, tomato paste, and seasonings. Cover and microwave on high $3^1/_2$ to 4 minutes, stirring once. Set aside.

Spread ricotta evenly over pie shell. Top with meat sauce. Cover with
plastic wrap and microwave on high 6 to $6^1/_2$ minutes; sprinkle with mozzarella cheese. Microwave uncovered on high 30 seconds, or until cheese
melts. Makes 6 servings.

May substitute ground round; drain well after cooking.

**variety of raw veggies marinated in no-oil Italian dressing, sprinkled with
Parmesan cheese*

Nutritional profile per serving:
21 g carbohydrate; 23 g protein; 8 g fat;
29% calories from fat; 46 mg cholesterol;
349 mg sodium; 248 calories

Part 4

PREGNANCY MOANS, GROANS, AND QUESTIONS

22

THE "WHAT ABOUTS" OF
PREGNANCY

REMEMBER: THERE ARE NO SUCH THINGS AS DUMB
QUESTIONS—ONLY DUMB MISTAKES.

After you announce the news that you're expecting, an amazing phenomenon takes place. Suddenly, everyone from your hairstylist to your mother-in-law (who was knocked out during her delivery and couldn't breast-feed) to the twelve-year-old boy next door becomes an expert on pregnancy. Ever heard, "You're carrying high, so I'm sure it's a boy!"? Or, how about, "I was sick as a dog each time I was having a girl."?

My goal is to give you the ability to separate good advice from nonsense—and to provide expert guidance on how to be your best while pregnant, overcoming symptoms safely and naturally.

What About Backaches?

You may notice that your back begins to ache as your pregnancy advances. Most pregnancy backaches consist of low-back pain, because the narrowest part of your back (your waist) has to balance your growing uterus and the normally stable joints in your pelvis begin to loosen somewhat to make easier passage for the baby at delivery. You tend to compensate for this sense of being off balance by bringing your shoulders back and arching your neck, thrusting your belly forward. The result: a deeply curved lower back, strained back muscles, and often extreme pain.

Since backache is so common during pregnancy, here are ten suggestions for avoiding or minimizing backache:

1. *Maintain good posture.* Pretend there is a string running through your backbone and out the top of your head. Imagine being pulled up by the string. Align your head, neck, backbone, and pelvis. Feel yourself lift and straighten. Consciously straighten your alignment when you feel yourself slouch. Also, avoid tilting your pelvis forward.

2. *Avoid extra weight gain.* The more extra weight you put on, the more weight your back will have to balance. If you cut out fat-laden and sugar-filled foods, the weight you gain is more apt to be "healthy weight" that is more evenly distributed.

3. *Elevate your legs.* When you sit, elevate your legs to take the pressure off your back. Or bend your legs and support your feet on a footstool.

4. *Wear shoes that give your feet support.* Some heel height is actually better than no heel at all—just don't go over two inches.

5. *Avoid lifting.* If you have to lift something, make sure it's not too heavy and lift with your legs—not your back. Bend at your knees while keeping your back fairly straight, grasp the object, then straighten your legs to lift.

6. *Try to avoid carrying objects in your arms.* Weight in your arms only adds to the weight already out in front of you. Instead, carry objects down at your sides or use a luggage carrier or other wheeled tote. Better yet, ask for help!

7. *Exercise moderately.* Ask your physician about exercises to strengthen and maintain your back muscles—these will make a big difference both now and after baby! Walk, swim, or do any acceptable exercise for pregnancy that you can do comfortably. It can help your back.

8. *Avoid standing for long periods of time*—and if you must stand, do so with one foot elevated on a footstool.

9. *Support your sleep.* Sleep on a firm mattress that offers good back support.

10. *Warm up to pain relief.* Take a long, warm bath, morning and evening, and try applying a heating pad wrapped in a towel for up to twenty minutes, three or four times a day. Most of all, relax. Many back problems are aggravated by stress and tension.

What About Bladder Infections?

Pregnancy makes women more prone to bladder infections, and the longer the urine stays in the bladder, the more likely it is to grow bacteria if such bacteria are present. Common signs and symptoms of an infection include pain and a burning sensation when urinating, urinating frequently, or voiding just a few drops at a time.

These tips will help to prevent bladder infections, or to keep them at bay. Start at the first sign of symptoms.

1. *Drink plenty of water to flush out your system*—at least eight ounces every hour on the hour for at least eight hours.

2. *Be sure you're getting sufficient vitamin C*—go for oranges, strawberries, broccoli, and mangoes. Do not take extra vitamin-C supplements without speaking with your doctor.

3. *Reach for drinks high in acidity* (like citrus and cranberry juice)— Cranberry juice has actually been shown to reduce your chances of getting a bladder infection to begin with—it prevents bacteria from sticking to the cells that line the urinary tract. Choose a cranberry juice that is 100-percent juice, with no sugar added (such as Dole Cranberry White Grape or Mott's Apple Cranberry).

4. *You should already be avoiding main irritators and known offenders*— nicotine, alcohol, caffeine, and artificial sweeteners, but add chocolate and carbonated drinks to the list.

5. *Every time you urinate, be sure your bladder is completely empty*—leaning forward while you are voiding will help. And don't put off urinating—"holding it" can increase your risk of infection.

6. *If you are put on antibiotics, be sure to eat freshly fruited yogurt with active cultures to help restore your balance of the "good" bacteria.*

If the symptoms continue or increase, call your doctor that very day. If the symptoms are accompanied by chills or fever, call your doctor immediately.

What About Breast-Feeding Preparations?

You may have noticed that your breasts are changing a great deal to prepare for feeding your baby after birth. Your breasts will enlarge and become fuller. Tenderness is normal. Veins become more noticeable under the skin, and the nipple itself will darken and enlarge. You begin to produce a creamy-like fluid around the fourth month and may even notice some leakage. If so, just remove with warm water or gently rub it in—it makes a great moisturizer!

If you have chosen to breast-feed, begin now to prepare your nipples by exposing them to air and sunlight and by gently tugging and rolling them. You might try going braless around the house and sunning braless through a window. Don't wash your nipples with soap, and don't rub them with a towel to toughen them. Although advised at one time, "toughening" the nipples is to be avoided because it removes the skin's natural protective qualities and can cause premature labor.

Choosing a pediatrician who is all in favor of breast-feeding will also be critical. Your doctor's

ATTEND A BREAST-FEEDING INFORMATION CLASS; YOUR DOCTOR'S OFFICE OR THE HOSPITAL YOU HAVE CHOSEN MAY HAVE ONE. YOU MAY ALSO WANT TO ATTEND A LA LECHE LEAGUE MEETING. LOOK IN THE PHONE BOOK FOR THE LOCAL CHAPTER'S PHONE NUMBER OR CALL THE TOLL-FREE NUMBER ON PAGE 227 FOR INFORMATION. FIND A FRIEND WHO HAS BREAST-FED AND WHO IS WILDLY ENTHUSIASTIC ABOUT IT THAT YOU CAN CALL WHEN YOU HAVE QUESTIONS OR JUST NEED SUPPORTIVE WORDS.

position on feeding is an important criteria for choosing him or her as your baby's health provider.

Use the time before your baby comes to be sure you have nursing pads and a breast pump on hand. (I suggest a battery-operated pump rather than a hand pump—it works much better!) You will want to pack some pads to take to the hospital and have the breast pump ready for when your milk comes in.

What About Close Pregnancies?

Sometimes it's planned, often it is a serendipitous happening—but you can find yourself pregnant once more when your baby is still just that—a baby. It happened to me: Danielle, my first, was only seven months and nursing heartily when I discovered that Nicole was on the way. My dear friend Carolyn had two toddlers and a ten-week-old when she discovered that number four was coming in about eight months! We both delivered beautiful, healthy little girls, although we both felt a bit tattered ourselves!

Conceiving again before you've fully recovered from the last pregnancy and delivery puts tremendous demand on your body. Giving yourself the best of care, starting the moment you discover (or suspect!) you're pregnant is the goal—doing everything possible to meet your needs and those of your new baby.

The Healthy Expectations Meal Plan becomes a lifeline to be adhered to faithfully. Your body may not have rebuilt your nutritional stores yet—so some overcompensation becomes important. Pay particular attention to your protein, iron, calcium, and B-vitamin intakes.

If you are still toting some of the weight from the last pregnancy, don't let it become a fixation that puts you into a calorie-deprivation mind-set. This new baby needs the same weight gain of twenty-five to thirty-five pounds from you that his sibling did—so don't even think about trying to lose weight while pregnant. You can make this weight gain just as healthy as the first (or even more so, now that you're experienced!)—and lose it well after this delivery.

If you are still nursing, and if your child is older than six months, speak with your doctor about continuing. Trying to rally the nutritional forces to 1) meet your own needs, 2) meet the needs of the new baby developing within, and 3) meet the need of your nursing baby is difficult at best. I did continue nursing Danielle until nine months, three months into my pregnancy with Nicole, and it took tremendous planning and tremendous amounts of food!

You need almost supernatural rest—and it will be a supernatural move for you to get it! Enlist whatever help is available—lie down when baby is napping, have Daddy take over as many nighttime feedings as possible, and forget the house.

What About Complexion Challenges?

You may be thinking, *This is the worst case of acne I've had since my junior prom!*

It may even be your first breakout since high school, and it's not unusual. The rosy glow of pregnancy is not just a myth. It is the result of hormonal changes, increased circulation to the blood vessels in your face—and the sense of awe that you are "growing a baby." There are other skin changes that aren't a myth either and aren't so rosy. The same hormonal changes that bring that glorious glow of pregnancy through an increased secretion of oils may also bring about less-than-glorious breakouts! Or your generally healthy skin may become dry and itchy or darken in spots.

The darkening of your skin can affect all parts of your body. When it affects the forehead, cheeks, or upper lip, it is called the "mask of pregnancy." For most people, this will fade within the year after delivery, and there are medications that help more stubborn cases. Don't take extra vitamin C or E—as is often recommended— in excess. Both can be toxic to the baby. Women who get breakouts around their periods are a bit more apt to experience them in pregnancy, but no one is immune. Here are some suggestions to banish breakouts:

1. *Stay on track with the Healthy Expectations Meal Plan.* It will give your skin the nutrients needed for staying in proper balance. Make sure you are including whole-grain carbohydrates like brown rice or whole-wheat breads, cereals, and pastas. These are filled with vitamin B_6, a vitamin used to treat hormonally induced skin problems.

2. *Drink lots and lots of water*—it's one of the most effective pore purifiers around.

3. *Wash your face two or three times a day with a gentle cleanser like Cetaphil.* Avoid skin-clogging creams and makeups.

If your skin challenges get extreme enough to warrant a visit to a dermatologist, be sure to let it be known that you are pregnant—and continue to let it be known. Many treatments for acne, such as Retin-A, can be extremely harmful to your baby.

Beyond acne, dry, itchy skin may also be a problem. Follow the same tips above, particularly the focus on your water intake. Moisturizers will also be a great help, especially when applied right out of the shower while the skin is still damp. This provides the best absorption. In the winter, try to keep heated houses well humidified; be careful not to bathe too frequently, thereby increasing dryness of the skin.

What About Constipation?

Constipation is very common in pregnancy, especially during the early weeks and again toward the end. In addition to the pressure of your growing baby on the the bowels, pregnancy hormones are slowing the rate at which foods move through your digestive tract and decreasing the strength of its muscles. This can result in major problems with constipation and gas formation unless you help your gastrointestinal tract speed things up. Fiber and water act like a sponge in your digestive tract and help your food pass more easily.

Be sure to get plenty of whole-grain carbohydrates, specifically unprocessed wheat bran, fresh fruits, and leafy vegetables. Be sure to drink adequate water (eight ounces before and after every meal and snack). You might try filling a two-quart container with water each morning—be sure it's gone by bedtime.

Also, exercise, especially walking, on a daily basis will help keep the digestive tract moving. Just a fifteen-minute walk each day will do a world of good!

HEALTHY GOAL: LAXATIVES AREN'T A HEALTHY WAY TO GET RID OF ANYTHING; FIBER, WATER, AND EXERCISE ARE.

What is fiber?

Grandma used to say, "Eat your roughage." Now, years later, the surgeon general says, "Double your fiber."

Fiber is linked to the prevention of our killer diseases: heart disease, obesity, cancer, and diabetes. The time has surely come to start increasing its amount in the diet. This can be done rather easily, not with "fiber pills," but by increasing your intake of whole-grain breads and cereals, unprocessed bran, beans, fresh fruits, and vegetables. These foods not only provide fiber but many other essential nutrients that cannot be obtained from other sources.

Fiber is the part of plants not digested by the body. There are two types of fiber: The water-soluble fibers are found in oats, barley, apples, dried beans, and nuts; they have been found to lower serum cholesterol and triglyceride levels and to help control blood sugar levels. The water-insoluble fibers are found in wheat bran, whole grains, and fresh vegetables; they are an excellent means of controlling chronic problems of pregnancy—constipation and hemorrhoids.

Think of fiber as a sponge that absorbs excess water in the GI tract to curtail diarrhea, providing a bulky mass that will pass more quickly and easily to relieve constipation and diverticulosis and possibly prevent hemorrhoids. Fiber needs water to make it work the way it should, ideally eight to ten glasses a day. The best way to drink water is to have a glass before and after every meal and snack rather than with a meal when it dilutes digestive functions.

What does fiber do for me?

- Fiber increases in the diet have been found to lower blood pressure as much as 10 percent with no other dietary changes.
- Those population groups with high-fiber intakes have a low incidence of many different types of cancers, particular colon cancer.
- Fiber's bulky mass in the intestine promotes fullness. This, combined with the fact that high-fiber foods take longer to eat and stay in the stomach longer, keep you full longer.
- Fiber serves as a "timed-release capsule," releasing sugars from digested carbohydrates slowly and evenly into the bloodstream. This helps keep your energy levels even.
- Fiber helps to protect against heart disease by lowering your level of "bad" LDL cholesterol.

- Fiber regulates your pregnant, and thereby slow, GI tract.

How do I double my fiber?

1. *Use whole grains* such as brown rice, oats, and whole wheat rather than the white refined types. When purchasing, look for words such as "100 percent whole wheat" with the word *whole* first in the ingredient list. Many manufacturers call products whole grain even if they contain only minimal amounts of bran. Brown dye does wonders in making food look healthy.

2. *Eat vegetables and fruits with well-washed skins.* You do need to peel the ones with wax on them.

3. *Choose more raw and lightly cooked vegetables,* but in as nonprocessed form as possible. As a food becomes processed, ground, mashed, puréed, or juiced, the fiber effectiveness is decreased.

4. *Add a variety of legumes* (dried beans and peanuts) to your diet.

5. *It is important to choose whole-grain foods at home* to fill the void of what is missing in restaurants.

6. *Add unprocessed raw bran to your cereals.* Raw oat bran (from oatmeal) is particularly useful in reducing cholesterol levels; raw wheat bran is useful for a healthy, regular GI tract. Be careful to add bran gradually; begin with one teaspoon wheat bran and one teaspoon oat bran, and increase slowly as your body adjusts to more fiber. Both types of bran may be purchased from your grocery store.

....

HEALTHY GOAL: INCREASE YOUR FIBER TO KEEP YOUR GI TRACT REGULAR, TO HELP FIGHT KILLER DISEASES, TO KEEP FEELING FULL LONGER, AND TO HELP YOU SAY NO TO OVEREATING BY KEEPING YOUR BLOOD SUGAR LEVEL EVEN.

....

Good health is everyone's major source of wealth. Without it, happiness is very difficult.

What About Cravings?

Could you just kill for a chocolate-chip cookie? Although often dismissed as temperamental whimsies, an excuse for most women to indulge their appetites, cravings could be tied to more physiological changes. They've been thought to reveal a mild zinc deficiency or simply reflect the hormonal changes of pregnancy resulting in unstable blood sugars. The cravings get fueled by diet deficiencies: Fluctuating blood sugars—enhanced by stress and hormones—stimulate the driving desire for sweets, fluid imbalances drive the desire for salty foods, and sustained inadequate intake of calories (lack of supply to meet demands) fuel the desire for fats. This is the physical side of the craving, driving us in a general direction; the emotions play into the exact food we arrive at.

With the physical side of a craving, the body sends out the "I NEED" signal. In the emotional side, the emotions send out the "I WANT" signal—sending us toward the comfort food of choice, particularly when comfort is being called for. Our generation's battle cry is, "Relief is just a swallow away," and for many of us that spells food—the refrigerator light becomes the light of our life.

Cravings usually become serious business during the fourteenth to twenty-eighth weeks of pregnancy, the "golden days" when eating is most enjoyed during pregnancy. It's after morning-sickness tendencies have subsided and before the baby is taking up too much space to enjoy a big meal.

Sharyn, another one of my patients, told of the secret missions on which she would send her husband. He made nightly trips to fast-food restaurants for the biggest, gooiest burrito he could buy. The burritos had to be loaded with

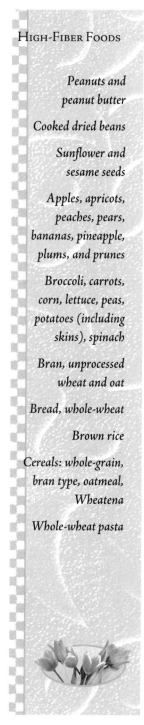

HIGH-FIBER FOODS

Peanuts and peanut butter

Cooked dried beans

Sunflower and sesame seeds

Apples, apricots, peaches, pears, bananas, pineapple, plums, and prunes

Broccoli, carrots, corn, lettuce, peas, potatoes (including skins), spinach

Bran, unprocessed wheat and oat

Bread, whole-wheat

Brown rice

Cereals: whole-grain, bran type, oatmeal, Wheatena

Whole-wheat pasta

hot sauce, beans, cheese, and guacamole to satisfy her craving for spicy Mexican food. Every night she would vow to be over her cravings, but every night they would seem to overtake her! The problem was that heartburn was overtaking her as well—and she needed to get some control back. We developed a meal plan that more completely met her needs, and her cravings came into check. For Sharyn, like most of my patients, it was all a matter of eating right foods at right times throughout the day to control her hunger of the nights. Smart eating throughout the day keeps the cravings crunch away!

Should you ever give in to cravings? Honestly, in pregnancy they are almost a homicidal drive—just try to stop you! The goal is to try to prevent them by keeping blood sugars stable, nutrient and fluid needs met—and if they happen, to make the best of them.

If you crave ice cream, go for frozen sorbet and yogurt with fresh fruit. If it's chips—go for baked chips and salsa, with a string cheese for protein. Don't try to analyze too much at the time; just make the best choices you can and figure out the "whys" later.

What About Depression?

Mood swings are more than normal during pregnancy—they are a way of life! They may be at their greatest, and you may be at your lowest, during the first trimester.

Avoiding excess sugar intake, chocolate, and caffeine (all of which will bring you up only to let you *down*) will help. But your best defense is to follow the Healthy Expectations Meal Plan, particularly focusing on eating often throughout your day. This will help to stabilize the chemical gymnastics your hormones are putting you through and keep you from falling off the high bar! A good balance of rest and exercise will also make a world of difference, as you'll benefit from the feel-good chemicals that are released. Read more about dealing with the emotions of pregnancy in chapter 23, "The Many Moods of Waiting."

Also talk with a friend, counselor, or pastor. Just talking through your feelings and anxieties can allow the brick wall around your emotions to come tumbling down. That's important, because depression is often just "frozen emotion."

You are experiencing one of the biggest transition periods of your life—and many emotions, both positive and negative, will rise to the surface. Processing these emotions is vital to your emotional—and physical—well-being.

What About Exercise?

Keeping active while you are pregnant can be as beneficial to you psychologically as it is physically. Most woman find that exercise reduces the aches and pains associated with pregnancy and boosts their energy levels and self-esteem. Labor and delivery are stressful and require a lot from your body. It will be more comfortable for you if you have good muscle tone, and exercise increases your stamina to endure the labor. In addition, research suggests that regular moderate exercise may reduce a woman's risk of developing two of the most dangerous illnesses associated with pregnancy—gestational diabetes and preeclampsia. That alone is reason enough to get in gear with fitness. But add this as well: You will probably get back into shape faster and more easily after delivery if you've kept your body in good condition during your pregnancy.

Regardless of whether you exercised before becoming pregnant, there's no reason why you can't begin a moderate program (with your physician's approval). During pregnancy, special consideration is needed for fitness; a pregnant woman is physically different.

During normal pregnancy, maternal blood volume increases about 30 percent, and heart rate and cardiac output are significantly elevated. The increased blood volume, coupled with the additional weight gain, causes a pregnant woman to reach her target rate with less vigorous activity than when not pregnant.

Excess heat should be avoided; specifically, avoid hot tubs, whirlpools, or steam rooms because they heat up the body's core temperature much more quickly. In addition, if you live in a

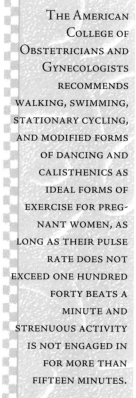

THE AMERICAN COLLEGE OF OBSTETRICIANS AND GYNECOLOGISTS RECOMMENDS WALKING, SWIMMING, STATIONARY CYCLING, AND MODIFIED FORMS OF DANCING AND CALISTHENICS AS IDEAL FORMS OF EXERCISE FOR PREGNANT WOMEN, AS LONG AS THEIR PULSE RATE DOES NOT EXCEED ONE HUNDRED FORTY BEATS A MINUTE AND STRENUOUS ACTIVITY IS NOT ENGAGED IN FOR MORE THAN FIFTEEN MINUTES.

city where pollution can build, avoid exercising outdoors when levels are high. Neither you nor your baby need to be deep-breathing pollutants.

Most doctors place restrictions on exercises with a high risk of falling, such as horseback riding, skiing, and skating. Sports involving balance may increase risk during pregnancy because of the altered center of gravity. Also avoid any work so strenuous that it competes with the baby for oxygen. Don't exercise flat on your back after the first trimester as it can decrease the blood flow to the uterus. Also, don't stand motionless for long periods. Ask your doctor for the body-building exercises specifically recommended during pregnancy for muscle strength and flexibility.

Workouts don't have to be elaborate, just regular. In fact, a gentle walking program and some basic stretching can be the first step toward a lifetime of fitness. It's something we all know how to do, we can do anywhere, and the only equipment we need is a comfortable pair of shoes. Many pregnant women have reported that their appetites decrease, they sleep better, and their general sense of well-being improves after making walking a part of their daily routine. Exercise and good nutrition are a dynamic duo for a healthy pregnancy!

Another great exercise choice in pregnancy is aquatics. In addition to the buoyancy, you get the advantage of the resistance of the water (about twelve times that of air) to gain strength and enhanced aerobic conditioning. Instead of pushing iron, you're pushing H_2O!

Whatever your choice for exercise, the goal is to maintain a fitness level you feel good about. If you exercised before, refuse to compare yourself to how fit you were before. Don't let workouts become a stress! You don't have to be the fitness queen—remember that you're supporting two bodies now, and it's natural to tire more easily. Admire your body for its abilities to do what it is doing rather than becoming frustrated at what you can't do.

The bottom line on exercise is this: If your body is tired, listen to it and rest. If you are obsessing on exercise, you really may be obsessing on trying to take control back. Your body is changing rapidly, your emotions seem to be spinning out of control, and you may be frightened about giving birth. Or you may feel incapable of being a mother or, at least, a good one. Excessive exercise can give you a sense of getting a grip—but it's grasping the wrong thing.

Exercise is no guarantee for shorter deliveries or healthier babies.

But it is a sure bet that you'll feel better, you'll be healthier, and your body will not feel quite as though it's playing the lead role in "Invasion of the Body Snatchers!"

You may experience small uterine contractions during or after aerobic exercise, but this is normal. You should stop exercising if it causes bleeding, painful cramping, nausea, or shortness of breath. Discuss any problems with your doctor. If you are already involved in a fitness program, you should consult with your physician about any guidelines he would like for you to follow.

Reasons Not to Exercise

- Pregnancy-induced hypertension (high blood pressure)
- Preterm rupture of membranes
- Past experience with preterm labor
- Persistent bleeding during the second or third trimester

Stop exercising if you experience:

- Dizziness, faintness, or shortness of breath
- Irregular or rapid heartbeat
- Pain, especially in your back or pubic area

Training Tips

- Always include Kegel exercises at least three times per day (see page 174 for explanation of Kegel exercises).
- Don't exercise in hot, humid weather or when pollution levels are high.
- Wear well-cushioned shoes that provide good support.
- Wear a bra that fits properly and supports your breasts well.
- Drink water before, during, and after every workout.
- Tilt pelvis to a neutral position and squeeze shoulder blades together to avoid overarching your back.
- Begin each exercise session with five to ten minutes of low-intensity exercise such as walking. Complete your warmup or cool down by stretching calves, chest, lower back, and hamstrings. Hold each stretch for twenty seconds without bouncing. For cool downs, increase the stretch time to thirty seconds.
- When walking, walk as if you were wearing a crown—your ears

should be centered over your shoulders, and your shoulders should be over your hips.

- After the first trimester, avoid doing any exercises in a flat-back position. The weight of the baby can affect blood flow to your brain, making you dizzy. If you begin to feel lightheaded, slowly roll over on your left side until the feeling passes. Then sit up.

Kegels: A Powerful Exercise—Pregnant or Not!

Kegels are a miracle exercise and easy to do. You should do Kegel vaginal exercises daily—aim for ten to twenty-five repetitions two or three times a day. To do Kegels, firmly tense the muscles around your vagina and anus, as if you are stopping the flow of urine. Hold for as long as you can, working up to eight to ten seconds, then slowly release the muscles and relax.

- Do Kegels either before or after every meal.
- Practice them as you shower and when you brush your teeth.
- Do a set when you're stopped at a red light or waiting to pay a toll.
- Exercise those pelvic muscles to the rhythm of your windshield wipers.

What About Fatigue?

"I'm *so-o-o* tired!"

It would be surprising if you weren't tired! In some ways, your body is going through the stress and demands you'd experience if you were running a marathon—you just aren't able to count off the miles!

The fatigue you feel in early pregnancy is often the worst kind—it can be compared to being on double doses of nighttime cold medicine all day long. The hormone hurricane you are in causes blood sugars to swing wide and wild, causing energy to drop and often to stay low. In addition, the hormonal changes cause chemicals to be released that keep you in a constant search for a couch, any couch, anywhere! Generally this exhaustion will lift as you move into the second trimester. But sometimes it doesn't, and that's when it becomes important to take a closer look.

Of course, fatigue can stem from more elusive factors such as stress, sleep problems, anemia, or something as simple (yet little known) as not drinking enough water. More often the likely cause is something predictable—simply being underfed and underfueled and unable to perk up. You may not be getting enough rest, or you may be overcome by the stresses of living life and growing a baby—all at the same time. Particularly in the first trimester, when the body is manufacturing your baby's entire life support system along with adjusting to the vast physical and emotional demands of being pregnant, fatigue is a natural.

By the fourth month, your body will be adjusted and energy will begin to pick up—but until then, and even after, give yourself a break! You may need to work fewer hours or sleep more. Be sure to follow the stressbuster tips on the next page—avoiding the energy robbers. Double-check to make certain that you're meeting all your needs (compare your diet to the Healthy Expectations Meal Plan on page 84). Fatigue is often a sign of a deficient intake of protein, iron, and calories. No matter how tired you are, don't be tempted to reach for what seems to promise a quick boost. Caffeine, candy bars, and soda won't fool your body for long—and after a quick lift your blood sugars will bring you down *hard*. This will leave you even more fatigued.

If this is your first baby, enjoy what may be your last chance (for a long, long time!) to focus on taking care of you without feeling guilty. I can't tell you the number of times after I had two babies under two that I looked back on those first days of pregnancy and wished I had taken afternoon naps when I had a chance.

Keep your evenings free of unnecessary activities, and get yourself out of the need to have your house perfect. (It will be great training for after baby!) Spend time off your feet reading, journaling, thinking of baby names, and connecting

THE POWER OF THE AFTERNOON NAP CANNOT BE OVERSTATED. JUST TWENTY MINUTES OF SLEEP CAN DO MIRACLES FOR REGENERATING THE BODY. IF YOU CAN'T SLEEP, JUST LIE DOWN (REMEMBER, ON THE LEFT SIDE!) WITH A GOOD BOOK. IF YOU ARE AT AN OFFICE, USE YOUR BREAK TIMES AS A TIME TO SIT QUIETLY WITH YOUR FEET UP ON A DESK OR RESTING IN THE LADIES' LOUNGE. IF YOU ALREADY HAVE CHILDREN, DISCIPLINE YOURSELF TO NAP WHEN THEY NAP—AND TO IGNORE THE LAUNDRY.

with those you love. If you have older children, this is a great time to read to them, play quiet games with them, or supervise their cooking for you.

Expect fatigue to return a bit in the last trimester—it may be God's way of slowing you down and storing every dab of energy for the big event! Take the opportunity to let others pamper you. If they ask what they can do to help, *tell them!*

If fatigue is severe or accompanied by fainting, heavy perspiration, breathlessness, and/or heart palpitations, discuss it with your physician. It may be time to do a check for anemia; it is certainly cause for an all-points check.

How to Recharge Instantly

You won't have to wait for these stressbusters to take effect. They'll revive you right away:

1. *The shoulder shrug.* While sitting or standing (or riding on a subway) raise your shoulders as high as you can, reaching for your ears. Hold them in that position for a few seconds and then drop them to their normal position. Repeat three times. Benefit: You'll instantly relieve upper chest and shoulder tension.

2. *The "rag doll."* Stand with arms dangling loosely at your sides and start to shake your hands. Then start shaking your arms. Next, sit and repeat the same moves with your legs. You'll feel less tense and more alert in minutes.

3. *The natural lift.* Getting outdoors can recharge you in a flash. But even gazing out the window briefly may do the trick. Studies show that patients recovering from surgery have less pain and fewer complications if they have a view of trees from their room.

4. *The TV turn-off.* That's right—switch off the TV. It may surprise you, but although television seems relaxing, research shows people feel less relaxed and less satisfied after watching TV than they did before.

What About Frequent Urination?

"I can't stay out of the bathroom! How can I possibly urinate this often?"

It's not your imagination—you probably are doing aerobic-level bathroom trips! It's also not abnormal. . . .

One of the reasons for the increased urinary frequency is the increased volume of body fluids as your kidneys become much more efficient. Another is the pressure of your growing baby on the bladder. This pressure is somewhat relieved around the fourth month when the uterus rises somewhat, higher up into the abdomen area. But the pressure returns in the ninth month, when the baby "drops" into position for birth.

Be sure to empty your bladder fully each time you urinate. This is helped by leaning forward when you urinate. If your sleep is being interrupted by middle-of-the-night bathroom trips, try drinking your day's intake of water by 5:00 P.M. Don't limit the water—you and your baby desperately need it! Just control when you drink it. Also be sure that you're getting enough protein, evenly eating it throughout the day. This will ensure proper fluid balance.

What About Gas—Bloating and Flatulence?

Why does it happen in a crowded elevator? No one knows, but what brave researchers tell us is that the average nonpregnant Joann passes gas fourteen times each day. You can expect to pass even more when pregnant! It doesn't mean something's wrong—excess gas production is just a natural by-product of a slower movement of food and waste through the system. It can also be aggravated by what you eat or by your lifestyle.

To diminish these winds, try these tips:

1. *Limit the main gas-producing foods:* melons, cabbage, cauliflower, corn, broccoli, Brussels sprouts, iceberg lettuce, legumes. You don't have to avoid them, but eat them at different times and in smaller portions, or de-gas them by sprinkling on an enzyme mix like Beano.

2. *Chew your food and dine slowly.* Gulping food means gulping air, which ultimately looks for a noisy escape! The more slowly you eat, the less air you swallow, and

ALTHOUGH AGGRA-
VATED BY CITRUS
JUICE, TOMATO
SAUCES, CAFFEINE,
PICKLED FOODS,
CHILI POWDER,
PEPPER, AND
PEPPERMINT CANDY—
HEARTBURN IS
CAUSED BY THE
HORMONAL CHANGES
OF PREGNANCY AND
THE MECHANICAL
PRESSURE OF THE
BACK PUSHING
AGAINST THE GASTRIC
AREA. HORMONAL
CHANGES DURING
PREGNANCY CAUSE
EMPTYING TIME IN
THE STOMACH TO
SLOW, WHICH, IN
TURN, CAUSES THE
SPHINCTER BETWEEN
THE ESOPHAGUS AND
THE STOMACH TO
STAY MORE RELAXED
THAN NORMAL,
ALLOWING THE ACID
IN THE STOMACH
TO BE FORCED BACK
INTO THE ESOPHAGUS.
ALL OF THESE
CHANGES MAY
CAUSE HEARTBURN.

the better your food is broken down, so the less likely you are to suffer from gas. Take time when you eat, and don't wash food down with water. Instead, drink your water after your meals and snacks.

3. *Exercise!* It helps to get your bowels on the move and prevents gas from getting—and staying—trapped. Walking can do wonders to relieve that bloated gassy feeling!

4. *Stay away from sugarless gum.* The sorbitol, a natural sweetener used in sugarless gums and candies, is a major gas former.

5. *Avoid going more than two-and-one-half to three hours without eating,* allowing acids to build to explosive levels.

6. *Drink water after meals and snacks, not on an empty stomach.* Cut out the carbonation.

What About Heartburn and Indigestion?

You feel like you're on fire. Your insides are burning—you feel pressure under your ribs and an acid taste in your mouth. You have heartburn—a most unpleasant yet all too common sensation of pregnancy.

Heartburn can be controlled by eating in an evenly distributed way throughout the day, helping to keep gastric acids neutralized. Do not resort to antacids! Remember—eat to prevent heartburn rather than trying to treat it once it's started.

Here are some ways you can cool the heartburn:

1. *Eat* very *often*, eating balanced mini-meals every two to two-and-one-half

hours to keep the gastric acids neutralized.

2. *Steer clear of heartburn aggravators:* caffeine, pickled foods, chili powder, pepper, and peppermint candy. Orange juice and tomato sauces are major problems for many and are the first things to avoid if heartburn is chronic.

3. *Slow down your eating and* dine. Heartburn may be caused by eating too fast. We aren't just a fast-food generation; we're a fast-eating one, too.

4. *Trim the fat from your diet*—and excess sugar, too. Both sugar and fat aggravate the burn.

5. *Be sure to drink lots of water*—but after meals, not on an empty stomach. Even water can cause an acid explosion if there is no food in the stomach to neutralize it.

6. *Be careful not to gain too much weight*—the baby is putting enough pressure on the area. Don't add fuel to the fire!

7. *Sleep with the head of your bed elevated six inches.*

8. *Don't wear clothes that are tight around your waist,* and avoid bending over at the waist.

If all else fails, do talk to your doctor about a low-sodium antacid or other reliever that is safe for pregnancy. I've worked with many a pregnant mom who enlisted Tums as her after-dinner mint!

What About Hemorrhoids?

Hemorrhoids are swollen blood vessels in and around the anus and lower rectum, the equivalent of varicose veins in your legs. They are more apt to develop in pregnancy because of the pressure of the baby on the abdomen and the hormonal changes that cause the blood vessels in the rectal area to enlarge. Hemorrhoids can cause itching, pain, even rectal bleeding.

Use these tips for prevention of hemorrhoids:

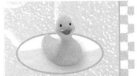

FOR RELIEF FROM HEM-
ORRHOIDS, TRY THE
FOLLOWING:

1. Warm sitz baths twice a day. *Fill your bath with three to four inches of warm—not scalding-hot—water. Add nothing to the water—oils, bubble bath, even Epsom salts can irritate the area. Lie back in the tub for thirty minutes if you can. Or do this for less time, more often. Let it be a moment to relax as well.*

2. A dab of witch hazel works wonders. *Take a cotton ball, soak it in cold witch hazel, and apply it against your hemorrhoid until it's no longer cold; then repeat. Ice packs can also be quite comforting.*

1. *Don't get constipated.* Preventing constipation completely is the best way to prevent hemorrhoids completely. Drink lots of water, increase your fiber, and exercise. Don't strain when having a bowel movement.

2. *Lie on your left side for about twenty minutes every four to six hours.* By doing this, you decrease pressure on the main vein draining the lower half of the body. Also avoid long hours of standing or sitting—both put pressure on rectal veins.

3. *Do Kegel exercises regularly*—they increase circulation to the area. (See page 174 for more information on Kegels.)

Use topical medications, suppositories, or stool softeners only if prescribed by your doctor. *Do not use mineral oil.*

If you are experiencing rectal bleeding, try not to self-diagnose this as hemorrhoids. It could be, but it could also be the sign of something more serious. Rectal bleeding should always be evaluated by your physician. However, if hemorrhoids are the diagnosis, take on the starring role for treatment. Self-care is the ticket to eliminate discomfort and the need for more radical measures.

What About Herbal Remedies?

Don't make the mistake of thinking that although you can't take many medications while pregnant it's safe to use natural herbal remedies—just because something is "natural" does not mean it is safe. Herbs are drugs—often very powerful ones and quite harmful to you and your baby. Some can cause miscarriage—others can cause diarrhea, vomiting, and heart palpitations.

An added risk with herbal medicines is that they are not manufactured under the same quality-controlled conditions as traditional FDA-approved medications, thereby having variable strengths and possible contamination.

Remember that just because something is natural and made from plants does not make it automatically safe. Some herbs, like arnica and pennyroyal, can cause uterine contractions or diarrhea to you and can be toxic to your baby. Ginseng contains steroid-like properties and should be avoided.

Just treat herbal remedies as you would any drug during pregnancy. Simply do not take them unless directed to do so by your doctor. Even herbal teas should be used cautiously. While some herbal teas, such as raspberry and ginger, are considered safe and natural remedies for upset stomachs, when you are pregnant only choose a commercial brand such as Lipton or Celestial Seasonings, which are under federal regulations and scrutiny. Sometimes the problem with herbal brews is found in their unsafe processing.

If you have symptoms that need treatment, seek the advice of your practitioner—do not self-treat, and don't listen to your Aunt Susie!

What About Holidays and Parties?

There is nothing like the holidays to bring out the best of our memories—and the worst of our eating habits. Being pregnant during this time can be a big challenge to work through—especially when you are focused on eating according to the Healthy Expectations Meal Plan.

Here are survival tips for remaining alive, well, and merry in a world that overeats and most often eats unhealthily:

1. *Always eat a healthy snack before going to parties* so that your "appetite for the appetizers" will be in control!

2. *Don't try to starve on the day of a big party!* You will only slow down your metabolism and set yourself up for a gorge because you will be so hungry. Instead, eat

smaller, evenly spaced meals throughout the day.

3. *Remember that it's not the "big parties" that are a problem—but the day-by-day eating.* Eating well in between the "big days" will help to stabilize your body. Avoid the "I've-blown-it-now" syndrome and let each day be a new beginning.

4. *Try to make the focus of parties more than just the food itself.* Plan other activities besides eating! Games are fun for everyone and give a new direction from the usual gorge. Talk to friends in rooms other than where the food is served.

5. *Never tell people you can't eat something—doing so is self-sabotage!* You will instantly be a candidate for being talked (or badgered) into everything! If you feel you must say anything, just say, "I am not hungry quite yet." Don't look pitiful in a corner! No one ever notices that the life of the party isn't eating.

What About Itchy Tummies?

"My belly itches constantly—it's driving me nuts!"

It's quite simple—pregnant bellies are simply itchy! As your baby grows, the skin across the abdomen stretches tightly. The result is dryness, causing intense itching. Try not to scratch—it can cause the area to become inflamed, even infected, and result in unwanted scarring. Do try lubricating lotion (such as calamine), or "milk it down"—dip a washcloth in cold milk and apply it to your skin for five minutes. Milk has anti-inflammatory properties that often take the itch away. In addition, it contains lactic acid, which is very soothing.

The best time to moisturize is right after a bath or shower while you're still damp and your skin is plump with moisture. Moisturizer will help to lock in the natural moisture so that it doesn't evaporate.

Take warm—not hot—baths using a very mild soap such as Dove, Lever 2000, Tone, or Caress.

What About Leg Cramps?

They seem to hit in the middle of the night—and they are very painful. Muscle cramps, or charley horses, can take your breath away. They can be caused by many things: the slowing of your blood circulation, the pressure of the baby's head on certain nerves, and possibly a calcium/magnesium imbalance or a potassium deficiency.

Nothing feels better than to lie down and stretch out pregnant muscles! Often, this stretching means extending your feet away from you. And it does feel great, until the charley horse hits! *Not* stretching in that way is one thing you can do to prevent these leg muscle cramps—and you can often get relief in the middle of one by sitting or lying down and flexing your toes and ankles towards your face. Push down on your knee at the same time to straighten your leg. Doing this several times with each leg before you go to bed may also help to ward off the leg cramp. Try elevating your legs on a pillow for sleeping.

If your baby is taking more calcium from you than you are receiving from your diet, you may be more prone to muscle cramps. Prevent this by boosting your calcium intake (see "What Are High-Calcium Foods?" on page 55) and by getting extra insurance against cramps from a glass of milk and a banana before bed. This bedtime snack gives valuable potassium, along with a boost in serotonin for better sleep.

Leg cramps are most common in the second and third trimesters, and fatigue seems to increase their frequency. Give your legs a break by wearing support hose during the day, and take the load off by resting frequently throughout the day with your feet up. Care during the day often has payoffs in prevention at night!

What About Moms Over Forty?

If you are over forty and pregnant, you are not just growing great with child, you are in good—and growing—company! The pregnancy rate in your age group is soaring—even for women having their first child.

One of the challenges you will have to face is listening to the warnings of cautious and caring health-care providers. As an expectant mom over forty, you will hear more than you ever wanted to know about chromosomal deficiencies and prenatal testing due to the increased risk for Down's Syndrome to your baby. Be aware that although there are increased risks in some areas, you *can* reduce risks in other areas. By putting your focus on getting the best prenatal care, practicing terrific self-care through diet, exercise, and rest, you can take years off your risk profile, making your chances of delivering a healthy baby as good as those of a much younger mother.

You do need to be careful to avoid the "Superwoman Syndrome," as you may already have many responsibilities on your shoulders—more than what a twenty-two-year-old may have. You may have an established career, teenagers, or aging parents requiring care—or all of the above. Getting enough rest in your pregnancy is critical; you deserve it! Don't wait until your body starts pleading with you to slow down.

It takes careful planning to get enough calcium into your body to both provide for the baby and protect you from your age-increased risk of osteoporosis. After age thirty-five you need five servings of high-calcium foods each day—with pregnancy added in, you need six servings, or an equivalent amount (eighteen hundred milligrams) through supplementation.

What About Multiple Births?

No one can begin to track the intense and wide gamut of emotions that are experienced with the news of a pregnancy. The news of "more than one" is just that much more powerful!

The physical needs of a multiple-birth pregnancy are powerful as well. The requirements for vitamins and minerals increase, with a particularly high need for iron, calcium, and folic acid. A supplement of these is usually given in addition to the prenatal vitamins and minerals. The mom expecting twins—or more—needs to learn all about preventing anemia (see page 57) and should increase her intake of high-calcium foods to six servings each day. She should also eat lots and lots of dark green leafy veggies.

Energy demands are particularly high with a multiple-birth pregnancy, so the need to eat evenly and properly throughout the day and evening is very important! Rest is also vital—definite rest periods with Mom lying on her side will be prescribed early in the pregnancy to avoid early labor. An extra serving of carbohydrates and one more ounce of protein should be added to each meal in the Healthy Expectations Meal Plan (page 84), and two glasses of low-fat milk or its equivalent should be added as a snack. Eating every two hours will also keep the appetite in better control.

When the pitter-patter of little feet becomes a stampede, how much weight should I gain?

The total weight gain should be thirty-five to thirty-seven pounds for twins and thirty-eight to forty pounds for triplets. Following the Healthy Expectations Meal Plan each day, but letting your appetite guide you for portions, will help you keep a proper weight gain, stamina, and energy. I generally add an extra serving of protein to each meal and snack—and an extra serving of carbohydrate to each meal.

What About Prenatal Multivitamin and Mineral Supplements?

If you follow the recommended nutritional guidelines and make healthy choices, the chances are that you will get the vitamins and minerals you need during pregnancy. However, because you may eat on the run or occasionally make unwise choices—or may even be too sick to eat—your doctor may have prescribed a prenatal multivitamin/multimineral supplement for you to take. The supplement will fill in the needs you may not have met that day, but don't let your prenatal vitamin and mineral supplement give you a false sense of security that you don't have to be concerned about your diet. No supplement can ever replace food as your source of nutrition. No supplement is divinely created. There are many substances in food that are just being identified as vital for a healthy pregnancy and thereby just now being included in a prenatal supplement. For example, zinc wasn't found in prenatal supplements twenty years ago, but whole-wheat bread has always contained it.

To sum it up, don't believe that you can take a vitamin supplement to replace good food, and don't believe that poor eating can ever be solved by a pill.

Take your supplements as directed and be sure not to medicate yourself with additional dietary supplements. Never take a supplement without your doctor's advice—pregnancy is no time to experiment! Many vitamins and minerals, if taken in additional megadose quantities, can seriously harm you and your unborn precious child. Your baby's liver, the organ that breaks down or stores extra vitamins, is still underdeveloped, and needless nutrients may circulate for a long time, causing tissue and organ damage.

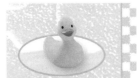

A COLD OR MILD ILLNESS DURING YOUR PREGNANCY MAY BE UNCOMFORTABLE, BUT IT WON'T HARM YOUR BABY. HOWEVER, SOME OF THE MEDICATIONS YOU MAY NORMALLY TAKE (LIKE DECONGESTANTS AND ANTIHISTAMINES) COULD. SO DON'T TAKE ANYTHING—EVEN EXTRA VITAMIN C—WITHOUT SPEAKING TO YOUR DOCTOR. YOUR DOCTOR CAN GIVE YOU THE MOST UP-TO-DATE LIST OF THE MEDICATIONS THAT ARE KNOWN TO BE SAFE—AND THE PROPER DOSAGE FOR THE SYMPTOMS YOU ARE EXPERIENCING.

Consistent high doses of vitamin C could make your baby dependent on it, requiring unusually high amounts of vitamin C after birth that can't be met through normal feeding.

You may feel that your prenatal vitamin seems to cause, or add to, the nausea in early pregnancy. If so, with your doctor's advice, try switching brands to get a different formula. Taking the supplement after meals will help, and so does taking it at night with your bedtime snack. I've even had some very nauseous patients open the capsule and sprinkle it into their fresh fruit shake.

You may also find that the iron in the prenatal supplement may cause stomach cramping or constipation. Switching formulas may help here as well—or the best choice may be taking a supplement that has no iron, and then adding a separate supplement of ferrous gluconate. Ask for advice.

HEALTHY GOAL: TAKE YOUR PRENATAL SUPPLEMENT AS PRESCRIBED. BUT REMEMBER: JUST BECAUSE A LITTLE IS GOOD, MORE IS NOT NECESSARILY BETTER!

What About Sickness?

It's one thing to get hit with the sniffles and a miserable cold if you are not pregnant—it's awful when you are pregnant and don't have a lot of options for treatment. So, what do you do?

The good news is that some of the best remedies for cold and flu symptoms are naturally safe for you and baby. Try these:

1. *Use a commercial saline spray preparation or a solution of one-fourth teaspoon salt in eight ounces water.* Put a few drops (or sprays) in your nose, then wait five to ten minutes and blow your nose. If your throat is sore or scratchy,

increase the salt in the saline solution to one teaspoon to eight ounces of hot water and gargle for five minutes. Repeat every two hours. The warm liquid and salt can help shrink and dry mucous membranes.

2. *Drink lots and lots of water, at least eight ounces every hour.* Also try hot fluids, like chicken soup. If you enjoy spicy foods, and can tolerate them, the heat can boost your immune system. Garlic works wonders as well!

3. *Use lots of steam.* A humidifier, a steam vaporizer, a steaming kettle (used with caution), or sitting in the bathroom for fifteen minutes while a hot shower runs will also heal your sinus passages, shrinking them and keeping them moist and less bacteria friendly.

4. *Alternate hot and cold compresses if there is a progression to painful sinusitis*—it may help. Dip a cloth in hot water, wring it out, and apply to the painful area until the heat dissipates, about thirty seconds. Then apply a cold compress until the cold dissipates. Continue alternating heat and cold for ten minutes, four times each day.

5. *Slather on a mentholated rub.* Rubbing your chest with an aromatic rub like Vicks can really make you feel better and less congested.

6. *Never starve your cold, your fever, or you!* Keep eating small, balanced meals often throughout the day according to the Healthy Expectations Meal Plan. Force yourself to eat if you must; try some of the fresh fruit shakes for a refreshing treat to sip on at mealtimes.

Most of all, REST! Try to get to bed, or at least get extra rest, at even the first symptom of a cold to prevent it from blossoming into a doozy.

Speak with your physician before taking any cold medication—over-the-counter or otherwise—and if you start running a fever.

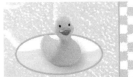

What About Sleeping: Getting a Good Night's Rest?

If you find yourself waking up during the night or sleeping restlessly, be sure that you have a bedtime snack that will keep your blood sugar levels more even as you sleep. It will keep you sleeping more deeply and will prevent a lighter state of sleep that acutely makes you aware of baby aerobics, full bladders, and general discomfort. An ideal snack is a whole-grain cereal with skim milk or yogurt. Also, try to drink most of your water intake before dinner—not afterwards.

The lowered metabolic rate of the first months of pregnancy may result in an increased need for sleep. You should attempt to get at least eight hours of sleep a night, and don't feel guilty about taking a short nap during the day; this will not be easy to do once the baby arrives. You may find your sleep patterns changing in the final months, as many women seem to require less sleep. Listen to your body and understand that adequate rest is a major part of wellness.

As you get bigger, getting comfortable in bed becomes a challenge. Lying on your abdomen is not comfortable, and sleeping on your back may leave you feeling dizzy, lightheaded, and nauseous due to the effect of the growing uterus on the heart's blood-pumping action. What's left? Here are some suggestions:

1. *Sleep on your left side.* This is the ideal position for circulation—particularly if you are retaining fluids in your ankles and feet. Tuck one or both knees up slightly and place a bed pillow between them. As the baby and your tummy grow, you may want to rest your belly on a pillow as well. In this position, you can maximize blood

flow to the baby and reduce swelling in your legs. You can alternately turn to the right side, but it is not as effective on snoozing on the left.

2. *Sleep in an easy chair.* If your bed just isn't working, try reclining in an easy chair with your legs propped up on an ottoman. You may need to shift your body slightly to the left side.

Every night before bed while I was pregnant, I listened to praise music and recorded my feelings in my journal. Thinking about reading those feelings to my grown-up little one one day was an incredible thought with which to go to sleep.

What About Smoking During Pregnancy?

There are plenty of reasons to stop smoking—even when not pregnant—but there are many more when you are planning a pregnancy or discover that you are pregnant.

Fortunately, there is no evidence that any smoking done before pregnancy—even if it's been for years—affects the development of your baby. But once pregnant, particularly after the fourth month, smoking is an extreme hazard to your little one growing within. The urine of newborns whose moms smoked has the same levels of nicotine as that of adult smokers.

Smoking lowers the amount of oxygen that reaches your baby, and it may also reduce the amount of nutrients available to the baby from the placenta. Studies show that there are two-and-one-half times more premature births and three times more low-weight babies born to smoking mothers. Smoking has also been associated with increased risk of miscarriage, stillbirth, placental bleeding, and possibly lower IQs in children. Behavioral problems are more prevalent in the sons of moms who smoked while pregnant. In addition, smoking by either parent is related to a higher risk of childhood cancer for a child.

And don't forget: If you stop smoking now, you will be providing a home for your baby to be born into that is free from smoke. Infants of smoking parents tend to come down with more respiratory illnesses. Be kind to that precious baby and make its home, both before and after its birth, a healthy place to be.

Happily, the Center for Disease Control and Prevention reports that the number of women who smoke in pregnancy continues to decline—down to 14 percent in 1995.

Any time a pregnant mom quits smoking she will reap immediate benefits—but it has been shown particularly beneficial if the nonsmoking status begins by the fourth month. It may be easier to stop smoking in the first trimester of pregnancy than at any other time, when a sudden distaste for cigarettes and cigarette smoke often arises. The body's protective mechanism may be working perfectly as it was created—if you are blessed with such a natural aversion, take advantage of it! If such a natural aversion doesn't show up, you may need to enlist the help of "Smoke Enders" or another smoking cessation group. Ask your doctor for a recommendation.

What About Stretch Marks?

They are lines on your skin that look like runs in your stockings, except you don't wear stockings where they are! They are stretch marks, and it is largely a matter of heredity as to whether or not you get them. About 90 percent of all women will develop stretch marks at some time during their pregnancy.

The best news about stretch marks, even if they show up on you, is that they fade to a silvery-white color after birth and really only show up in the sun.

Again, good skin tone, good skin elasticity (encouraged by good nutrition), and gradual (not rapid or excessive) weight gain can prevent or minimize stretch marks. There are several massage oils, lotions, and creams on the market that boast results, but they don't really seem to help prevent anything but skin dryness, no matter what the the product claims or how much you pay. They may make you feel good, smell good, and take the itchiness of the stretching tummy away—but they haven't been found to prevent the dastardly marks.

What About Swelling?

Swelling, or edema, is normal during pregnancy and is caused by the increased amount of fluid in your bloodstream. It's more noticeable in the ankles and feet because the baby's weight puts pressure on the veins in your pelvis, slowing down the flow of blood from the legs to the heart. At times, however, the swelling may seem excessive and may cause a sudden, unexplained jump in weight. In nonpregnant women, fluid retention is often caused by too high an intake of salt. In pregnancy, excessive swelling is more often caused by inadequate protein intake. Be sure you are eating two ounces of high-quality, low-fat protein every two to two-and-one-half hours throughout the day! Although salt used to be a no-no for pregnant ladies, we now know that excess fluid retention is not usually caused by a normal salt (sodium chloride) intake; in fact, you require some sodium during pregnancy! Don't restrict your fluid, don't take a diuretic (unless your doctor prescribes it), and don't cut out all sodium.

Watch the Salt

The chemical name for salt is *sodium chloride*—with sodium being the more important in terms of health. The highest concentrations in foods are in cured ham, bacon, pickles, potato chips, and cold cuts where the sodium is used as a preservative.

Excessive sodium is indicated in many diseases, especially hypertension (high blood pressure) and kidney disease. Excess salt causes temporary buildup of body fluids in your system. This makes it difficult for your heart to pump blood through the cardiovascular system, and the results may be high blood pressure or excessive swelling.

The taste for salt is conditioned, and as you begin to use less of it, your taste will change so that you will enjoy foods more with less. Be patient with yourself and your family. Gradually cut back on its use in cooking, and cut out completely

EVERYONE REQUIRES SOME SODIUM, AND, ALTHOUGH YOUR NEED FOR IT DURING PREGNANCY ACTUALLY INCREASES, THERE'S MORE THAN ENOUGH SODIUM NATURALLY PRESENT IN FOODS TO SUPPLY THIS REQUIREMENT. SODIUM SHOULD NOT BE SEVERELY RESTRICTED DURING PREGNANCY, BUT IF YOU USE SALT TO AN EXTREME, IT WOULD BE WISE TO CUT BACK ON ITS OVERUSE. BECOME AWARE OF WHERE YOU MAY BE USING SALT IN EXCESS. MOST OF US CONSUME FIVE TO TWENTY-FIVE TIMES MORE THAN WE NEED.

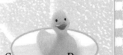

Seasoning Blend 1

2 tsp. dry mustard
1 tsp. garlic powder
1½ tsp. oregano
1 tsp. curry powder
1 tsp. marjoram
½ tsp. onion powder
1 tsp. thyme
½ tsp. celery seed

Combine all ingredients, mixing well. Store in airtight container.

Seasoning Blend 2

1 Tbsp. garlic powder
1 tsp. pepper
1 Tbsp. dry mustard
1 tsp. basil
1 Tbsp. paprika
½ tsp. thyme

Combine all ingredients, mixing well. Store in airtight container.

those snack foods that are triple threats: high in salt, fat, and calories. If you are directed to cut back on your sodium intake, here's how:

1. *Cut back on your use of more highly processed foods and salty snacks.*

2. *Leave the salt shaker off the table.* You'll quickly start enjoying the natural flavor of your foods without covering them with salt. Try substituting herbs and spices for some of the salt.

3. *Attempt to cook with seasoning blends rather than salt*—it will add new, exciting flavors to your cooking. Try making your own and keep them in a large-holed shaker right by the stove where your salt used to be.

4. *Try to limit your intake of these high-sodium foods:*

- Any food pickled or brine-cured, like sauerkraut and pickles.
- Any food salt-cured or smoked, like ham and bacon.
- Salted snack foods, like salted-top crackers and chips.
- Condiments, like soy sauce and ketchup. Use in moderation.
- Convenience foods, like frozen dinners and instant soup mixes.
- Most canned foods, like canned soups, vegetable juice, and canned vegetables. Check labels for sodium content.

Try some of the meals on pages 136–158; they will give you a chance to cook and enjoy foods without the usual added fat and salt.

Cheer up! Sodium does not have to be cut out completely; you only need to be aware of its sources and cut back on excess use. Accept the challenge of learning to cook and enjoy foods without the usual added fat and salt. Included in Part 3 are many wonderful recipes that are a great place to start.

And, if you do start to swell, try rest, rest, rest! Lying on your side or sitting with your feet propped up also helps.

What About Teenage Moms?

The pregnant teenager has an extra-special need for healthy food due to the extra-high demands pregnancy places on her body.

The teenage years are a time to complete growth and development and to rebuild body stores of nutrients used during the changes of puberty. This rebuilding time will continue for four years after menstruation begins. Becoming pregnant during this time will put the body at high risk for health problems because the nutrient stores will not be replenished. There is a greater risk of delivering a premature, unhealthy, or underweight baby as well as a greater tendency for the mom to develop toxemia and anemia. Read page 57 for the nutritional strategy to prevent anemia.

Eating the right thing at the right time can make the difference! It is a time to throw off the erratic dieting of teenage years and to focus on healthy eating. The pregnant teenager needs to eat for her still growing body as well as for the baby. She must be very careful to eat good whole-grain carbohydrates balanced with two to three ounces of protein every two-and-one-half to three hours throughout the day and evening. She will need five servings of high-calcium foods each day and lots and lots of those darkly colored fruits and vegetables (six servings a day), with two servings each day that are high in vitamin C.

HEALTHY GOAL: TEENAGE MOMS HAVE A LOT TO GAIN FROM A GOOD DIET—AND A LOT TO LOSE FROM A BAD ONE! REALIZE HOW CRITICAL IT IS TO YOU AND THAT SWEET BABY YOU ARE NURTURING TO EAT IN A HEALTHY WAY.

What About Toxemia?

Toxemia, or preeclampsia, is a condition found only in pregnancy; it consists of swelling, elevated blood pressure, and the loss of protein in the urine. The cause is not fully understood, but it appears that women who enter a pregnancy obese, underweight, or malnourished are more likely to develop the symptoms. It only occurs in 7 percent of first pregnancies and even less in later ones.

The symptoms usually appear about halfway through the pregnancy and could be related to inadequate protein or vitamin B_6 intake. If you develop toxemia or extreme swelling, be sure to pay special attention to the protein you are eating. Good sources of protein are listed on page 26; remember to have it every two to two-and-one-half hours with a whole-grain carbohydrate all throughout the day and evening. If a risk for toxemia is identified in one of my patients, I will aim for more than a hundred grams of protein each day in a mom's diet.

Although sodium is not the main culprit, it can aggravate the condition. Thereby you should carefully avoid excessive salt intake. Bed rest is vitally important; resting one to two hours each day on your left side will greatly help with the swelling as well as your feeling of well-being.

HEALTHY GOAL: DURING THIS TIME OF GREAT NUTRITIONAL NEEDS, CARE-FULLY FOLLOW THE HEALTHY EXPECTATIONS MEAL PLAN (PAGES 82–85).

What About Travel?

Traveling is stressful in the best of times—even if you're on your way to a week in the sands and sun of the Caribbean. It's not unusual to arrive at your destination exhausted, irritable, and feeling swollen and bloated. Since that pretty much describes being pregnant, traveling while great with child is a double-whammy stress. (Just think of Mary on the donkey!)

Use these tips to travel and stay alive and well—to ensure that you stay energized, strong, and safe:

1. *Let your star twinkle!* It pays to be vocal about your pregnancy when you travel—you may just find yourself

bumped up a class of service or invited to the front of the bathroom line. Especially if you're not showing yet, let flight attendants know; they empathize and will really try to attend to your special needs when possible.

2. *Drink plenty of water, especially if you fly.* A dry airplane cabin is ten times more arid than the Sahara, causing you to lose fluid through your skin. This leads to dehydration, which results in puffy hands and ankles, fatigue, and a generalized bloated feeling—again, pregnancy defined! The key for preventing the jet-plane blues is to drink eight to twelve ounces of replacement fluids each hour you are in the air. The best fluids: water, sparkling water or club soda, and fruit juices. The worst are those you are avoiding anyway: caffeinated drinks (like coffees, teas, and sodas) and alcoholic beverages. They intensify the dehydration.

3. *Order a special meal on airline flights.* Airline food is traditionally high in fats and salts and low on nutrition. Avoid it by requesting a dietetic meal when you book your flight or within twenty-four hours of your flight. There is no extra charge, yet the meal will be packed with higher fiber, lower fat, and real nutrition.

4. *Pack your own supply of power snacks*—see page 19 for those that do not need refrigeration. These snacks will allow you to keep eating the right foods at the right time—even with the challenges of travel.

5. *Wear comfortable clothing and shoes.*

6. *If you have a layover between flights, use the time to exercise.*

7. *Request an aisle seat,* so you can get up and stretch— keep moving! More than likely, the many trips to the lavatory will ensure this—but do try to move about the cabin every hour or so. If you are driving, short stretch breaks are also vital.

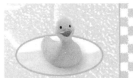

TAKE TIME FOR SOUL CARE. WHETHER YOUR TRIP IS FOR A DAY, A WEEKEND, OR A WEEK, LOOK FOR AN OPPORTUNITY TO GET AWAY FROM THE NORMAL DISTRACTIONS OF LIFE— LEAVE SOME TIME TO REFLECT ON THE MANY CHANGES TAKING PLACE WITHIN AND MAKE SOME SIGNIFICANT SPIRITUAL CONNECTIONS.

8. *Check your bags!* This is no time to be lifting carry-on bags, unless you have someone to carry them for you.

9. *Step out of jet lag.* When changing time zones, your pregnant body will thank you if you exercise within the first twelve hours of getting to your destination. When you fly east, take a gentle walk in the morning sun. When flying west, walk in the late afternoon sun. It helps your body adjust and will reward you with better sleep and more energy.

10. *Prepare for altitude changes.* If you're headed to the mountains, and you're used to living in lower places—make sure you're ready for the transition. It is sure to bring the enjoyment of your trip to a higher level! The decreased oxygen in the air at higher altitudes can cause headaches, breathlessness, fatigue, nausea, and disturbed sleep, and it can stress you and your baby. Discuss this with your doctor before you plan any trips to the high country!

Avoid the altitude stress by starting your trip slowly, moving to higher levels gradually, and attempting to rest a day after arriving to help you get adjusted. Eating your small meals of carbohydrate and low-fat proteins every two to two-and-one-half hours and drinking lots of water is critical. Get medical help if needed, but help yourself to some smart self-care!

Remember: If you are traveling outside of the

United States or after your sixth month, talk to your physician before making the reservations!

What About Varicose Veins?

Varicose veins are a common side effect of pregnancy. The extra volume of blood that your body produces to support the baby as well as the extra weight put pressure on the blood vessels in your legs.

Varicose veins can be prevented or their symptoms minimized by wearing support pantyhose, elevating your legs when you are sitting, avoiding prolonged standing, avoiding excessive weight gain, and exercising (in moderation) thirty minutes a day. Gentle aerobic exercises like walking, swimming, or exercise-biking will divert blood from the venous system back toward the heart. This is very helpful.

As your pregnancy advances, you may notice veins beginning to bulge. You'll want to guard against the pain and discomfort by continuing to wear support stockings, gaining no excess weight, elevating your feet when you can, moving your ankles while sitting, and continuing to exercise to improve blood flow.

Don't get too concerned about spider veins; most will disappear within six weeks of your delivery.

When your husband asks what he can do for you—be prepared to tell him—a foot rub! It relieves stress and tension, and it feels great.

What About Vegetarians?

The vegetarian diet can be a wonderfully nutritious and well-balanced way of eating during pregnancy. It is especially easy for a "lacto-ovo-vegetarian" (one who eats dairy foods and eggs), as the proteins in this diet are high-quality substitutes for meat and fish.

The pregnant "vegan" (one who avoids all animal products) must take special care in planning her diet to get enough calories and to combine plant proteins properly to get all the essential amino acids (grains with legumes or seeds with legumes). See the list of protein sources on page 26. Don't just rely on meat substitutes; some are very good protein sources, but others are low in quality protein and high in fat and calories. The vegan should also be sure that her prenatal supplement includes B_{12}; it is not present in plant foods.

The vegan will also have to put *major* focus into getting adequate calcium, something that is much easier for the vegetarian who includes dairy products. Many soy products are fortified with calcium, but not all, so become a careful label reader. Tofu is only a good calcium source if it has been coagulated with calcium—again a matter for careful label reading. In addition, I ask my patients who can tolerate citrus to drink high-calcium orange juice. And I usually have to move toward supplementing at least a part of the calcium demand.

Getting proper amounts of high-iron foods must be a priority for both types of vegetarianism. A consultation with a registered dietitian may be advised to aid in the careful planning of this special diet for a perfect pregnancy.

What About What to Take to the Hospital?

You will want to have a delivery bag and a suitcase all packed just waiting for when you go into labor.

Many hospitals want you to bring the following items:

- A pillow or blanket that reminds you of home—it will make you feel better!
- Two bras (nursing bras if you plan to breast-feed)
- Robe and slippers
- Nightgowns
- Small amount of change for incidentals
- Personal items (toothpaste, toothbrush, cosmetics, hairbrush, deodorant)
- Reading material
- Watch or clock
- Power snacks, especially Trail Mix
- The baby's "going home" clothes

Note: Don't take a lot of money, credit cards, or jewelry.

Your Delivery Bag

It's best to have a separate bag ready and waiting to take you throughout labor and delivery. This will not only be packed with necessities for you, but for Daddy as well. Your labor may be short, or it may be long, but it will definitely feel like a marathon event.

Although not easily packed—you may want to take a female friend along—accompanying you and Daddy to the birth. You can't imagine how helpful it is to have another person to "share the load" of caring for you through delivery. Research has even shown that the presence of such a dear friend promotes healthier and less painful deliveries. It's particularly helpful if your sweet friend has a good sense of humor. Laughter, even in the most difficult of situations, can boost endorphins, which diminish pain. More than likely, Dad may be feeling anxious and fearful—and that goes double for your mother—such emotions won't do great things for your own sense of well-being. Call and reserve that special person right away!

What About When to Call the Doctor?

Many of the unpleasant symptoms of pregnancy are simply that, symptoms of pregnancy with only one cure—delivery! That is why learning what you can do to prevent them from occurring or, at the least, how to relieve the discomfort takes you light-years ahead in enjoying this miraculous time.

However, there are certain symptoms that could be the sign of something serious occurring in your body or with your baby. Call your doctor immediately if you experience any of the following:

- Severe lower abdominal pain on one or both sides that doesn't subside, accompanied by bleeding, nausea, or vomiting.
- Heavy vaginal bleeding (especially when combined with abdominal or back pain).
- Coughing up blood.

THE DELIVERY BAG IS FILLED WITH ITEMS TO MAKE YOUR TIME AS COMFORTABLE AS POSSIBLE: LIP BALM, TENNIS BALLS FOR YOUR BACK, TRAIL MIX FOR YOUR HUSBAND (EVEN A SANDWICH, IF YOU HAVE TIME TO PACK ONE!), BOTTLES OF WATER, CHANGE FOR THE TELEPHONE, A LIST OF NAMES AND PHONE NUMBERS OF PEOPLE TO CALL, THE LONG-DISTANCE CREDIT CARD OR NUMBER, AND READING MATERIAL.

- A gush or steady leaking of fluids from the vagina.
- Fever over 102 degrees.
- Swelling or puffiness of hands, face, and eyes accompanied by headache or vision difficulties.
- Fewer than ten movements of the baby per hour after twenty-eight weeks.

Call your doctor within a day if you experience any of the following symptoms that do not subside:

- Severe upper mid-abdominal pain without nausea, bleeding, or vomiting.
- Slight vaginal spotting.
- Bleeding from nipples, rectum, or bladder.
- A sudden increase in thirst or urination, or no urination at all for an entire day.
- Swelling or puffiness of hands, face, and eyes with no headaches or vision difficulties.
- Severe headache that persists for more than two or three hours with no swelling or puffiness of hands, face, and eyes.
- Painful or burning urination, yet no chills or fever over 102 degrees.
- Severe nausea or vomiting (more than two to three times per day in first trimester) without fever or chills.
- Absence of noticeable fetal movement for twenty-four hours after the twentieth week.
- Overall itching.

The symptoms to watch for in pregnancy should be one of the first things you discuss with your doctor on your very first visit. Be sure you discuss when to call the doctor and what to do if you can't connect. What is the emergency plan?

If you call the doctor, be very specific about your symptoms and mention any other symptom you may be experiencing—even if it seems unrelated to you. Describe how long the symptoms have been experienced, how frequently they are occurring, if anything has relieved them, and how severe they are.

Remember, there are no such things as dumb questions—only poor answers and dumb mistakes. If you don't understand, ask again and again and again.

23

The Many Moods of Waiting

People who tell you they sleep like a baby
probably don't have one.

The awe and wonder of the positive pregnancy test may be quickly replaced by "What have we done?" This is no reflection on your love and commitment to your baby—it is just a reflection on the shake-up to your emotions that happens with pregnancy. There are hormone changes, body changes, relational changes, financial changes—every arena of life is blasted. My friend Lisa describes it as a "big baby bomb" that went off and leveled everything normal in her life.

Whether this is your first, second, or eighth child, your life will undergo incredible change both with the pregnancy and with the baby's arrival.

In any change, there is gain and there is loss. And there is always grieving—a natural part of change. Becoming a mom is exciting, but it can be fearful and sad as well. We may grieve for the carefree life we are leaving behind, we may fear that we won't be able to handle a baby, we may even resent what it's doing to our body and life. Jenny was thrilled about the baby growing within her, but she wasn't so thrilled with gaining forty pounds and being constipated!

And then there are the other fears: Did I drink too much coffee before I knew I was pregnant? How about all those diet sodas and the artificial sweeteners? I cried for two months—did all those stress chemicals hurt the baby? Can I get through labor? What if I "have" to use medications to help? Am I eating enough fish for the baby's brain development? Is the fish I'm eating from polluted waters?

Fears can be the ugly side of pregnancy—the clouds that block the sunny days of anticipation. Fluctuating hormones fuel fretfulness, right along with the moodiness that let worries come in and chat a while.

Here's Margaret's story; it may sound familiar to you.

> Immediately following the first numbing moments of reality with a positive pregnancy test—I'M PREGNANT?!!!—came an overwhelming sense of being terrified. Not specific fears, just a general sense of panic that there was a baby growing inside me, and I would be eternally responsible for her—forever!

Later Margaret's fears became a little more intense and much more focused . . . surfacing at strange times and coming in waves. *Should I have used that nose spray? Why am I cramping? What if I get tired of the baby like people get tired of puppies?* And even more difficult fears to even speak of.

If there are any positives to fear at all, one of them is this: Thinking fears through can help you develop a healthy sense of attachment and responsibility for your contribution to your baby's well-being. Processing them can also help you to begin to see what you can affect and what you cannot change. This will be important for the rest of your life as a mom.

Talking about your concerns is a way to see them differently. Just getting them out of the whirlwind of your mind, out of the dark, can let you see them through the light and power of truth. Ask questions. Talk to friends. Journal. Pray.

These are the most common fears faced in pregnancy and a healthy dose of perspective on them:

The Seven Deadly Fears

1. *I'm scared that I may lose the baby.* Miscarriage is one of the most common fears during early pregnancy, especially if you've had difficulty conceiving, if you've had any bleeding or spotting, or if you've had a miscarriage before.

   Healthy Perspective: The odds are very much in your favor for carrying your healthy baby to delivery. Even if you've miscarried before, you have no higher risk than had you not, and even after two miscarriages, your risk for having a third goes up only slightly.

Miscarriage is not a woman's fault and not something that can be controlled. However, you will feel more at ease knowing you've done everything possible to assure that you are at your healthiest-best for pregnancy: eating and resting well, avoiding alcohol and drugs, and getting good medical care.

2. *I'm scared that my baby won't be normal.* A healthy, perfectly developed baby is on everyone's prayer list while pregnant, and nagging fears can stick around till every toe is counted and the baby's doctor gives the high sign. Nothing can rob the joy of the process of carrying your baby like the fear of birth defects that can almost take on a life of their own. One of the negatives of having so much information available about your baby's growth and development is that you can also read about every possible thing that can go wrong.

Healthy Perspective: Although this is the biggest fear of pregnancy, 97 percent of babies are born without birth defects. Your responsibility is to believe for a healthy baby and to take great care of yourself before and after conceiving. Diligently follow your physician's instructions for care and keep your appointments. They are making sure all is well and keeping an eye out for potential problems at the same time. Prenatal tests can help, but they can often bring forth new and different anxieties. Your goal is to educate yourself about available tests and discuss thoroughly with your doctor which ones you may need and why. Then you and the dad-to-be can make the decision as to which ones you choose to have.

3. *I'm scared that my body will never be same.* The

THE FEAR ABOUT YOUR BABY'S WELL-BEING ACTUALLY CONTINUES THROUGHOUT YOUR LIFE AS A MOM—BECAUSE IT SIFTS DOWN TO AN ELEMENTAL ISSUE OF PARENTHOOD: HOW OUT OF CONTROL YOU REALLY FEEL. LATER, IT MAY SURFACE WHEN YOUR FIVE-MONTH-OLD HAS AN EAR INFECTION—AND YOU CAN'T MAKE THE PAIN GO AWAY. IF THEY HURT, YOU HURT. MOTHERHOOD—MORE THAN ANYTHING IN MY LIFE—KEEPS ME FOREVER ON MY KNEES, CONFESSING HOW LITTLE CONTROL I HAVE AND LOOKING TO THE ONE WHO HAS IT ALL.

physical changes of pregnancy—weight gain, enlarged breasts, puffiness—can be terrifying to women who held a tight grip on their body size and weight before they were pregnant.

Healthy Perspective: You're pregnant—not fat—and there is a huge difference! The padding of pregnancy is all about body changes that provide for the growth of the baby—the increased size of the breasts, uterus, even the muscles to support it. Your healthy goal is to eat with the guidance of the Healthy Expectations Meal Plan, which will allow you to geep your weight gain within the recommended twenty-five to thirty-five pounds. Taking care of yourself throughout your pregnancy, including moderate exercise, will have a huge impact on the state of your body after the baby is born. Nursing initially helps to pull the uterus back to a nonpregnant shape and size, but breast-feeding will also keep a few extra pounds on to provide for milk production. It will take more than a week or two to have your body back to its normal best, but it did take it nine months to grow a baby!

4. *I'm scared that I won't be able to stand the pain of delivery.* Labor fears often escalate in the third trimester because it's impossible to know what to expect. Even though you have heard story after story of labor and delivery (even from people on elevators!), yours will be uniquely different. And therein lies fuel for fears. You may worry that you'll make a mess of the bed or start screaming at your husband—or the doctor.

Healthy Perspective: The number-one way to allay the fears of labor is to learn what to expect. Women who aren't prepared for the birth experience have more anxiety, which results in more pain, which brings more anxiety. Knowing the pattern of labor, what to expect in a contraction, and planning how to deal with it is the secret to a more positive birth experience—physically, emotionally, and spiritually. Giving birth to a baby is not just something to "get through."

Identify your source of strength and the times when that strength has been your bridge to survival. Think about some of your most difficult times and journal your responses. What helped you? Humor? Determination? Prayer? See yourself calling upon that strength in childbirth.

5. *I'm scared that I won't be a good mom.* Anxiety about the kind of

mother you'll be is very normal. Concerns about everything from being able to calm a crying child, to knowing what to do—and being able to do it—in an emergency, to feeding issues can plague a mom-to-be.

Expecting a baby stirs buckets of feelings, often bringing forth deep issues about your own mothering. If your image of your mom is that she was perfect in every way, you may feel that you could never even come close to being as good. If your mom had difficulties with some parts of mothering, you may be terrified that it's genetic and that you'll be just like her.

Healthy Perspective: Your confidence will grow as you learn more about how your baby is developing, how your child grows, and how to cope with the different stages. Read everything you can from credible sources and surround yourself by friends or a new mom support group.

You may find great comfort being around your own mother. As you are being prepared to become someone's mother as well, you may suddenly find her reasons for doing what she did fascinating. As your baby grows and your love for that baby grows, you will have a new understanding of how much your mother really must have loved you. (It will also help you understand why it's so difficult—even when you're an adult—to give up being obsessed with your well-being!)

6. *I'm scared that my husband won't always be here.* Pregnancy has a way of making even the most independent woman become strangely dependent on her husband, physically, emotionally, and financially—all increasing her fear of losing him to an illness, accident, or marital problem.

   Healthy Perspective: The odds of a sudden illness or an accident are extremely small, and the odds of your baby's daddy choosing to disappear are smaller still. Practical assurances can come through having him get a complete physical and being sure that he always wears his seatbelt—for you and the baby.

7. *I'm scared that I won't love my baby (or won't love this baby as much as the first).*
   Healthy Perspective: You will. Trust me. You will love this baby. And, if this is number two, you are about to experience a most amazing miracle of life—that the immense love you feel for your

*Philippians 4:7
**Proverbs 14:30

first baby is about to be multiplied to more than you could ever ask or think. No matter what you were told by your mom about you and your brother, you won't "love them the same"—you will love them uniquely, but just as much.

Overcoming Fear

Fears are a natural aspect of any kind of change in life—especially changes that are affecting every part of your life: physically, emotionally, relationally, spiritually, financially. Yet peace of mind can become more of a craving than ice cream and pickles. Fear stops controlling us when we see that, although we don't have total control or always get to choose our circumstances, we do have choices in how we respond to life's events.

Your husband will be a valuable source of support, but also spend time talking with women, pregnant ones if you can! They will affirm your feelings, because they are most likely feeling the same way.

Take time every day to reflect on your pregnancy—whether a few quiet moments in the bath or shower, the last few moments before slipping into sleep, or the few moments after awakening. Keep a journal. (I vote for this!) It's very important to think about and verbalize what you are feeling.

A Word About Journaling

If you are like me, you may feel hesitant about journaling. No time, no privacy, nothing to write about. Your time of pregnancy is a perfect time to lay those protests aside . . . you have a very focused subject to write about, a bursting dam of feelings to be felt, and an incredible opportunity to record a miracle.

As you begin to write, your self-consciousness

will fade, enabling you to write more easily the feelings, thoughts, and fears that flood your inner soul and spirit. You can write about your joys, regrets, hopes, inadequacies, exciting happenings, moans and groans, happy thoughts, or what the baby did that day.

I've used special journals I've been given as gifts, and I've used an inexpensive spiral-bound notebook, even my notebook computer, to journal. Whatever you use, the journaling vehicle is just the tool.

Ten or fifteen minutes of peace can recharge you to rise up to the challenges ahead in the day. Pull away from the demands for a few moments to process your responses and collect your thoughts. Close the door, unplug the phone, and sit quietly. Go outside and sit—in your car if need be! If your children are young, encourage them to rest with you in a dimly lit room. If they are older, explain that you need a few uninterrupted minutes for recharge. Read, reflect on the struggles of the day, and lift them up through prayer or journaling. With less burden you can soar through the rest of the day!

Moods-in-Waiting

Being pregnant can give you the feeling that you are losing your mind, or at least losing control of what little you may have had. Your emotions may go from crankiness to violent outbursts of temper to weepiness to sobbing. You may also be totally unaware of your moods, and if someone dares to suggest that you seem a little "bothered," their very lives may be at stake.

The best way to handle these "many moods of waiting" is to understand that the hormonal hurricane causes emotional whiplash—and you just aren't going to be normal for awhile. Period. It's not chronic craziness, it's just with you for a spell. This is not a time for drastic measures like quitting your job (or your husband!). Accept it and allow for it—and do what you can to take charge of the physical you, which, in turn, undergirds and strengthens the emotional you.

There are many women who are convinced that any pregnant woman who tells you that her pregnancy is the most fulfilling and awesome time of her life is simply lying or has serious psychiatric problems. You may agree right now—but you may change your mind at the first Johnson and Johnson commercial.

You will be at your "worst" emotionally if your blood sugars are left to roller-coaster all on their own. You'll be able to better ride the

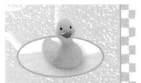

emotional tidal waves if you can stabilize the chemical gymnastics within before you fall off the high bar!

Wise eating, exercise, and rest will enable you to "stay afloat" rather than being caught in undertow of stress. Ironically, when life is most stressful, when we have the least amount of time or motivation to exercise, rest, and eat well, we need it most. I see this quite often in my pregnant clients and friends, unfortunately. When the stress realities of pregnancy come in their front door, wisdom about good eating choices can easily go out the window! It's easy to get distracted; the "eat-right prescription" can erode into "catch and catch can," and "quick and easy" can take precedence over nutritious. Energy plummets, leaving little motivation to exercise. An exhaustive cycle begins: The more stressed we are, the more unhealthy our eating becomes, the more guilty we feel, and the more stressed we get. The more stressed we get, the more fatigued we become, and the less stress-busting exercise we do, and the more we feel the effects of stress. It's not a pretty picture!

Although we know that healthy eating and exercise are more important now than ever before, they seem more like time-robbers and add to the already long list of "shoulds."

If this is a snapshot of your life, try turning the "shoulds" into "coulds." Taking charge of our choices is the one thing we can control—even in the midst of situations that feel out of control.

Choosing to follow the guidelines of the Healthy Expectations Meal Plan will provide a deflective shield against the symptoms of stress. It will gear up a stress-slowed metabolism, neutralize the stress-induced spurt of gastric acids, and stabilize digestive functions. As the blood sugars fluctuate in response to pregnancy hormones and emotional hurricane winds, the right foods at the right time will undergird them, keeping them even and high. When the body retains even more fluid than normal for pregnancy, adequate protein and fluid intake helps to restore fluid balance.

Properly timed and balanced eating will also energize you for exercise and allow for more restful sleep, both of which serve as swords at cutting away at the negative symptoms of stress.

Exercise is considered the key to responding positively to stress and change. This is why exercise is considered God's best tranquilizer. Gently exercising just thirty minutes a day is one of the best methods known for releasing tension. It can also be your quiet time in the midst of a busy, hectic day, a time when you can divert and reflect on your true source of strength.

There's only one other thing that cuts away at stress in a similar way as exercise and rest, and it is something to smile at—it's laughter!

It's so interesting to read what Solomon wrote about the subject—and to know that science now confirms it—"Laughter is good medicine."

24

Managing Miscarriage

MATURITY IS THE ABILITY TO LIVE AT PEACE WITH
THAT WHICH WE CANNOT CHANGE.

Though extremely difficult to accept at the time, when a miscarriage does occur, it is usually a natural process. Early miscarriage (within the first trimester) is generally the result of a problem in the baby's development. It may be related to poor implantation in your uterus, a genetic, chromosomal abnormality, an infection, or exposure to something toxic in the environment. The baby is just not able to survive.

Regardless, even knowing that "it was meant to be" and hearing the words "it is a blessing"—the process is still devastating. I know—my husband and I had a miscarriage just last year.

The pregnancy was an incredible miracle—and surprise! (Remember, I'm in my forties, with two teenage girls.) *I'm pregnant? Pregnant?* Those words seemed to be all I could say for weeks. The joy was of a fullness I had never experienced—and was like a tidal wave in our family. Really, it was as if our whole family were expecting—actually everyone who knew us—maybe all of Orlando! We saw the baby's heart beating—and I showed the sonogram on my TV show—announcing the wonderful news to the world.

And then at twelve weeks I miscarried, suddenly, one Sunday morning after a bit of spotting. It was as if my whole world came crashing in.

I was in perfect health, eating and exercising perfectly as well. I knew it wasn't my fault. But it hurt—it hurts—so much, more than anything I've experienced before.

If you have experienced the pain of miscarriage, don't look to place blame. It's not your fault—and it's not God's fault. Allow yourself to grieve, even though many people may not understand how deeply you are grieving. Share your feelings with your spouse, a dear friend, your pastor, or a counselor. Some communities have support groups for people who have experienced a loss in pregnancy. And it's not difficult to find another woman who has experienced miscarriage. It is so very common.

The best therapy recommended is to try to get pregnant again as soon as it is safe to do so. Discuss possible causes for the miscarriage with your physician before you do. If this was your first miscarriage, it was probably a random, one-time occurrence and is not likely to happen again. If you have had repeated miscarriages, there is a chance that your hormones are insufficient or that your immune system is running amuck with the signals. In these cases, treatment can prevent a miscarriage from recurring.

Take advantage of the recommended waiting period (three to six months) to focus on taking care of you—improving your eating pattern, establishing an exercise routine, and getting lots of rest.

And know that God is working all things together for good—that is a promise I have clung to over this past year, and it's for you as well. My ninety-five-year-old grandmother passed on at the end of this year. It was an incredible moment to know that she was joining the saints of heaven—and meeting my precious little one—as will I one sweet day.

Part 5

NEW LIFE—AFTER BABY

25

Feeding Your Baby— With Love and Good Sense

There are times when motherhood seems to be nothing but feeding the mouth that bites you.

Right up there with what to name your baby is the decision of how best to feed her. The decision to breast-feed or bottle-feed your baby is not one that can be made under pressure. It is your decision—and there is no wrong one. Read as much as you can about both so you can make the decision wisely. Your feelings will be sensed by your baby. This is your baby's most pleasurable time with you; make it enjoyable for both. The most important ingredient in feeding your baby is not what's given, but that it's given with love.

Bottle-feeding shares the love of feeding—especially with Dad. It gives you a break from the "Only You" song your baby sings in the middle of the night or throughout the day. And today's formulas more closely approximate the nutritional composition of breast milk, although they can't provide all the benefits of your custom-made milk. The formula you choose should be iron-fortified, and you should make the formula with purified water that contains fluoride. Discuss formula choices, including family history of milk or soy allergies, completely and thoroughly with your pediatrician before the baby is born. That's right, meet your pediatrician ahead of time to discuss these important topics.

With all the different viewpoints you'll hear, even the makers of these formulas agree about this: Breast milk is divinely created for

214

your baby. It is perfectly sterile and digestible. It is convenient (no formula or bottles to prepare); it's perfect nutritionally and is always the right temperature. It provides substances that give protection from infectious diseases and allergies, and it provides valuable omega-3 fatty acids that protect the body and even improve baby's IQ. Breast milk also makes baby less prone to constipation, diarrhea, colic, and gassy tummies.

Ninety-nine percent of women who want to breast-feed are physically able to do so. It does require time, patience, and a good sense of humor. The greatest period of adjustment comes during the first seven to ten days.

This adjustment time gets off to a great, or a hindered, start in the hospital. After the biggest accomplishment of anyone's life—delivering a baby—you aren't in a good strength position to be making decisions. This is why clearly knowing what you want to do regarding feeding your new baby is critical before labor starts!

Here are my suggestions; you may want to write them on a note-card and put them in your delivery bag:

1. *Let the delivery room staff know you are going to nurse the baby;* in addition to telling your doctor and nurses that you plan to nurse, have a note prepared to be placed on your chart. Tell them you want to breast-feed as soon as possible after delivery—either on the delivery table or in the recovery room. Nurse for five minutes on each side. The baby might just nuzzle, and that's fine—continue every one to two hours.

2. *Ask for "rooming-in" privileges with your baby to keep her with you for "on demand" feeding.* If you really would rather rest, knowing the baby is being well-cared for, have the baby brought to you frequently to nurse. Be sure the baby doesn't receive any bottles when she is not with you.

3. *Do not give supplemental water.* Make the nursery staff understand, and have it stated on the baby's chart, that they are not to give supplemental water—particularly sugar water—unless it is medically necessary for hydration. Unless a baby has a small birth weight and has

come through a stressful delivery, your colostrum is enough hydration. They have NO need for sugar water.

4. *Talk to the lactation consultant.* Ask to have the lactation consultant observe your nursing before you leave the hospital, and earlier, if you have challenges.

Many people find a great deal of help and support from the La Leche League, an organization dedicated to assist the breast-feeding mother. If you want to talk to someone when you're home, call your local chapter. They should be listed in your phone book. If not, call La Leche League International at 1-800-La Leche for your local contact. If you prefer to use your computer, visit their web site at http://www.lalecheleague.org.

Many hospitals now are staffed with a lactation consultant who can help you with nursing challenges, positioning for feeding, even tips for sore nipples! Ask if your birthing center has such a wonderful service, and use it—request a consultation before you leave for home and get names and phone numbers for help afterwards. You'll pick up great tips such as using olive oil as a moisturizer on your nipples to alleviate any cracking and soreness caused by nursing. It's not harmful to the baby, and it's great for you, three to four times per day.

The wonderful eating habits that allowed you to produce a healthy baby will allow you to produce healthy milk. If you are breast-feeding, you need to consume at least twenty-five hundred calories per day, which is approximately two to three hundred more than a good diet while pregnant. At full milk production, your baby will be taking eight hundred to one thousand calories from you each day and a quart of fluid. So eat, drink, and stay healthy!

You may have an incredible appetite during the first few weeks. Remember, you are recovering from a birthing marathon, you now have "room to eat," and you have milk-producing hormones that are on the hunt for fuel. Keep taking your prenatal vitamins and keep focused on the Healthy Expectations Meal Plan—adding in an extra power snack, preferably one including a high-calcium protein food (your need for calcium foods increase in breast-feeding to five servings a day) right along with the energy-giving carbohydrate. You may want to start your morning feeding for the baby by drinking a glass of milk or having fruit juice and cheese.

The key with the extra calories is what your body does with them—using them as fuel to boost your metabolism. This is why breast-feeding not only helps you to shed after-baby pounds more easily, the milk-making hormones help to burn the fat that has accumulated in the hips and thighs at the end of the pregnancy. Don't get too anxious to get it off, though—after the initial loss, if you are losing more than one-and-one-half pounds a week you're losing too much to keep up your milk production. Your calories cannot fall below eighteen hundred per day and still produce an adequate quantity.

If your weight loss slows down completely or stops, you may not be taking in enough calories for nursing, and your metabolism is slowing down to conserve the energy for its priority. Remember, you have to eat right foods, at the right time, and in the right balance.

Equally important to your milk production and letdown reflex is your fluid intake. You will need ten to twelve glasses of water each day. You may have to keep a chart; busy mothers forget fluids easily. Nothing will interfere with your milk production more than not getting enough fluid. Another tip is to take a sixteen-ounce glass of water with you when you sit down to nurse and sip on it till it's gone. You will also need an extra serving of high-calcium food, five total servings each day.

Don't let plans to return to work after baby cause you to choose not to breast-feed. Thanks to breast pumps, it's more than possible to work and nurse your baby. It does take planning—but the rewards are far worth the effort! Even if you choose to nurse for a short time, the benefits to your baby are so worthwhile!

If you work and want to keep breast-feeding, nurse your baby once—twice if possible—before leaving for work. While away, pump on your baby's schedule or when your breasts feel full (use breast pads to catch embarrassing leaks). You can store expressed milk in the refrigerator for up to eight days, or in the freezer for up to six months.

Nurse your baby as soon as your get home, and try to feed on the demand the rest of the day and on weekends. That will keep your milk supply replenished and maintain your special bond with your sweet baby.

If you choose formula feeding, or need to use bottles to feed your expressed breast milk, here are some tips to make bottle feeding special for everyone:

- If possible, get away from company at feeding times so you can focus totally on baby.

- Make eye contact with your baby and smile (as if you could help it).

- Don't prop the bottle up even though you may be exhausted. It's potentially dangerous, and it sends unhealthy messages about eating to baby.

- Get very comfortable—put on soft music—let this be a time out for you. It's nourishing for you and baby!

- Try to get baby ready for a snooze before feeding if possible. Try to get the diaper changed before feeding time; it will allow a peaceful transition into nap or family time.

26

GETTING IT BACK AFTER BABY

THE PROBLEM ISN'T THE <u>PROBLEM</u>—THE PROBLEM
IS MY <u>ATTITUDE</u> ABOUT THE PROBLEM.

Your Weight

As much as you may not want to hear this (if this is your second baby, you know this), you won't be back into your favorite jeans when you leave the hospital with baby. Your body took nine months to expand, and it doesn't spring back overnight. Actually, it will take three to nine months to shed all your weight and get back into your normal-best form. If you're breast-feeding, you'll probably hold onto a few extra pounds until the baby is weaned.

Whether you breast-feed or bottle-feed, the most important things you can do after giving birth are to heal, stay as healthy and energized as you can, and take the best possible care of that sweet baby. To fuel you for these vital jobs, you need the Healthy Expectations Meal Plan more than ever!

If bottle-feeding, keep on the Healthy Expectations Meal Plan quantities for at least six weeks before cutting back. Remember, you are healing a body that's been through the biggest change of your life. Don't eat less than twelve hundred calories a day, and stay hydrated. If you are breast-feeding, you'll need to continue to focus on getting enough calories (twenty-five hundred per day) to keep your milk production—and your metabolism—up and strong.

When to Exercise

If you kept fit while pregnant, you'll want to resume exercising as soon as you feel physically ready and your schedule with baby permits. Wise exercise can speed recovery from delivery and make you feel more energetic, as well as help you "get it back"—your body and your mind!

At one time, women were advised not to exercise until their six-week postpartum checkup. But depending on the difficulty and length of your labor and type of delivery, your physician may approve your starting back fairly soon. The better shape you stayed in during pregnancy, the more you will be able to do and the quicker your body will respond. And respond it does; you'll experience much less lower-back pain or achy legs and more restful sleep (when sleep is an option).

The payoffs are far greater than getting back into physical shape—your emotional well-being is at stake here as well. Women who get back into exercise postpartum report feeling much more stable and in control of their drastically changed lives.

A Baby Step in the Right Direction

Walking is the activity of choice in the first days after delivery—it's low impact and less likely to cause pain in the tender places. You can even get started in the hospital! Take it slow and gently and increase time and intensity gradually.

Swimming can also be a great after-baby exercise, but only after all bleeding and discharge cease. Cycling is even fine, once sitting feels comfortable again, and stationary biking can get you back into a routine that's not dependent on the weather.

Avoid all bouncing and hard jarring movements—and don't go all out with maximal exertion aerobically or muscularly until you've completely healed. That will be a minimum of six weeks postpartum. However, YOU MUST BE CAREFUL! Even after this recovery period, you still may have softness of ligaments, which can leave your joints susceptible to injury.

You can get back into your workouts even if you are breast-feeding, but you will need to plan your exercise time around the baby. Nurse right before you exercise so that your breasts won't feel so full and you won't leak. Be sure to wear a support bra, but not one that binds the breast so tightly that milk ducts become clogged, potentially leading to a painful infection.

Weight Loss Plan for Women (after weaning)

Breakfast (within 1/2 hour of rising)

COMPLEX CARBOHYDRATE: 1 slice whole-wheat bread OR 1/2 whole-wheat English muffin OR 3/4 cup cereal with raw bran added (begin with 1 teaspoon bran, gradually increasing to 2 tablespoons)

PROTEIN: 1 ounce part-skim cheese OR 1/2 cup nonfat plain yogurt OR 3/4 cup skim milk for cereal OR 1 egg (limit whole eggs to 3 times per week) or 1/4 cup egg substitute

SIMPLE CARBOHYDRATE: 1 small piece fresh fruit

Morning Snack

CARBOHYDRATE: 3 whole-grain crackers OR 1 small piece fresh fruit OR 1 rice cake or Wasa bread

PROTEIN:1 ounce part-skim cheese or lean meat OR 1/2 cup nonfat plain yogurt mixed with 1 teaspoon all-fruit spread

Lunch

COMPLEX CARBOHYDRATE: 2 slices whole-wheat bread OR 1 baked potato OR 1 whole-wheat pita bread

PROTEIN: 2 ounces part-skim cheese OR 2 ounces cooked poultry, fish, or lean roast beef OR 1/2 cup cooked legumes

SIMPLE CARBOHYDRATE: 1 small piece fresh fruit OR 1 cup non-creamed soup

HEALTHY MUNCHIE (OPTIONAL): raw vegetable salad with no-oil salad dressing

ADDED FAT (OPTIONAL): 1 teaspoon mayonnaise (or 1 tablespoon light mayonnaise) OR 1 teaspoon butter or margarine OR 1 teaspoon olive oil or canola oil OR 1 tablespoon salad dressing

Afternoon Snack

Repeat earlier snack choices

Dinner

COMPLEX CARBOHYDRATE: 1/2 cup rice or pasta OR 1/2 cup starchy vegetable

PROTEIN: 2 to 3 ounces cooked chicken, turkey, fish, seafood, or lean roast beef OR 1/2 cup cooked legumes

SIMPLE CARBOHYDRATE: 1 cup nonstarchy vegetable OR 1 small piece fresh fruit

HEALTHY MUNCHIE (OPTIONAL): raw vegetable salad with no-oil salad dressing

ADDED FAT (OPTIONAL): 1 teaspoon butter or margarine OR 1 teaspoon olive oil OR 1 tablespoon salad dressing

Evening Snack

1 small piece fresh fruit OR 3 cups light microwave popcorn

Free Items

raw vegetables, mustard, vinegar, lemon juice, no-oil salad dressing

Your Mind

After your baby is born, the pediatrician steps in with a plan of care. Your physician is watching for the right progression to your recovery from the delivery. But who's minding your mind? Who's assessing to see that even with everything in your world topsy-turvy . . . with no sleep and fatigue . . . massive hormone changes . . . and the incredible demands of caring for your little one—you are still able to hold it all together?

The first Sunday after I brought home Danielle, my first daughter, was Mother's Day. My mom came over for breakfast, and we opened sweet gifts and even sweeter cards. While reading my first-ever Mother's Day card I started sobbing hysterically. I cried on and off all day—for the next week.

I kept saying to myself, "The first few weeks of your baby's life are supposed to be the happiest moments of life—right? Well, why do I feel so blue?"

I wasn't alone. Many new moms—50 percent actually—experience "postpartum blues" for three or four weeks, crying a lot, feeling detached, and out of sync. My good friend, Alice MacMahon (the director of Florida Hospital's Center for Women's Health), warned me about it even before I left the hospital with my sweet Danielle. She told me that after nine nights without uninterrupted sleep, a woman was a candidate for insanity. I can't tell you the number of wee-in-the-morning times I thought of those words!

My emotional fountain didn't keep overflowing, but it does for about one out of ten women. For them, the "blues" can become a state of serious depression. Crying becomes a way of life; they have continual feelings of being overwhelmed and unable to cope—and these feelings don't go away. Professional help is vitally important in these instances, particularly when thoughts of harming oneself or the baby begin to surface.

The hormonal hurricane raging inside is the underlying chemical cause of postpartum depression, and the new, massive stresses of life add to it: The natural anticlimatic feelings that come after birth, the extreme demands of caring for this baby, the fatigue and sleep-deprivation, and the relative ease of not caring for yourself are all issues that must be confronted.

The hormones usually do stabilize, but not necessarily in six weeks. Continue to focus on the truth that you were pregnant for nine months, and it will most likely take another nine months to heal. As for your emotions, healing comes as you learn a new way of looking at life and living life.

Here are some suggestions to beat the Baby Blues:

Bust out of the "Superwoman Syndrome." You can't do it all.
Eat great foods for great energy.
Avoid caffeine, alcohol, and sweets. They lift you up only to bring you down.
Take time for YOU—care for you the way you care for others, even baby.

Break away when baby naps and get a power nap—just twenty minutes recharges!
Ask for help and stop trying to do everything yourself.
Believe you never heard the name "Martha Stewart."
You deserve time out and away from baby. Dinner out can do a world of good!

Break to communicate with your husband; he needs you, and you need him!

Look for other women with new babies and start a support network.

Understand that these are difficult days that do not last forever!

Exercise! It's a great way to relieve your stress and energize.

Strive for simplicity—don't try to do as much as the "old" you.

Rest and Recuperation

It seems quite bizarre that we have to learn how to rest, that we need practical instruction to do so. But we do, because women, trained from our own birth to be givers and doers, often find it difficult to make time—or take time—to give or do for ourselves. Getting by on fumes becomes a way of life. Diane, a recent new mom who homeschools four older children, identifies. "I used to laugh that I was a *human doing* rather than a *human being*. I don't laugh about that so much anymore. Is it because I'm over thirty with this little one or because I'm just exhausted?" Maybe a little of both!

Pay close attention to the warning signs of physical and emotional exhaustion: Low milk production, weepiness, easily picking up infections. If the warning lights are blinking, go to bed for one whole day. Literally lie in bed or in the sun, reading, dozing, allowing the baby to nurse at will.

Take an hour's soak in the tub. Beg your husband for a back and foot rub. Play relaxing music. If you have other small children, they can get into the swing of "Mom's Day Off"—something important that can be a lot of fun. It can be their time to babysit for you and the new baby.

Prioritize: Avoid answering the phone and taking responsibility for anything but your own rest and care, and care for the baby. Throw off the guilt about uncompleted household tasks and other "to dos." Your physical and emotional renewal is the priority!

The Pieces Back Together

When I think back to my days with two babies under sixteen months—I can tell you of many, many special moments. I can tell you of quiet times nursing Nicole while I watched her big sister, just a baby herself, sleeping so peacefully. I remember the awe and wonderment I felt.

I also remember the sense of being overwhelmed—having so much heart for my girls and yet massive tugs and pulls at that heart.

I still feel that way at times. I tell the story about a time when Nicole was playing sweetly with her favorite Disney stuffed special—Eeyore. Older sister Danielle, upon seeing it, decided it would be an excellent time to play with the anxiety-ridden donkey as well. She grabbed one of its legs while Nicole staunchly held on to the other. As they tried to wrestle it away from each other, there was a ripping sound and a flurry of flying styrofoam stuffing. Poor Eeyore was left lying on the floor with a split belly, looking very sad and forlorn indeed.

How many times have I felt just like poor Eeyore, pulled apart and torn by every conflicting demand and the many roles and responsibilities I'm called upon—and expected—to fulfill? It's a battle. The continual tug of conflicting roles and responsibilities—beyond those of being a new mom and the never ceasing demands of the baby, there are commitments to spouses, parents, friends, church, possibly employers, even self.

A few years ago, I came to a desperate time of needing it all to STOP. A story of a woman who was desperate, just like me, became a pivitol word for me. I read of this woman in the New Testament, in Mark 5:25–34. She was a woman, bleeding to death, who came for healing. This passage has rich promises for those of us who feel torn and fragmented by the demands of being a mother.

Think for a moment what it must have been like to be singled out by the awesome God of the universe when Jesus spoke to her, "Daughter, your faith has healed you. Go in peace and be freed from your suffering."* After years of frustration and hopelessness and a sense of bleeding to death, she found herself restored to health. In that moment I believe she received not only healing, but freedom from suffering—emotional, spiritual, and physical—as well. What a moment!

Too many times I felt just like her, as if I were bleeding to death. How about you? At times, does your spirit, your soul—as well as your body—cry out for wholeness? Mine did. In the fragmented midst of wearing this hat and that hat I needed to feel whole: complete, real, worthwhile, on purpose. I wanted to be sewn back together, not fragmented and torn at the seams like Eeyore.

*Mark 5:34

HEALTHY EXPECTATIONS

I am so thankful for this story of a woman whose simple faith teaches me to reach out for a loving, powerful touch. I find joy in hearing Christ's comforting words "Daughter, your faith has healed you"—because I know they are for me, and I believe they are for you.

Appendix:
Valuable Resources

The American College of Obstetricians and Gynecologists (ACOG) Resource Center. This organization will send information on pregnancy and women's health upon request. Please write: 409 12th Street, S.W., Washington, DC 20024-2118. Enclose a SASE along with your request. Or you may call (202) 638-5577.

La Leche League International. This organization can provide tremendous breast-feeding information and support. Call (800) LA-LECHE.

March of Dimes Resource Center. The March of Dimes provides information on prepregnancy and pregnancy, including genetic influence, lifestyle influence, and environmental hazards in pregnancy. Call toll-free (888) MODIMES.

Maternal and Child Health Center. This organization gives good information. Call (202) 625-8410.

National Center for Nutrition and Dietetics Consumer Hotline. This consumer hotline is a valuable source of nutritional information. Call (800) 638-2772.

Vegetarian Resource Group. This resource group provides great helps for living vegetarian. Call (410) 366-VEGE.

Recipe Index

Subject Index

Menstruation, 76, 193

Mental, 44, 60

Mentality, 68

Metabolism, 12, 52, 110, 188

Milk, 8, 13-14, 18-20, 25-28, 32,
34, 39, 44, 47, 55-56, 82-85, 87,
93, 95, 105, 107, 111-113, 115-
118, 123-124, 135, 148, 151,
164, 182-183, 185, 188, 204,
214-217, 219, 221, 224

Milk-producing, 216

Mineral, 7, 56, 58, 74, 105, 180, 185

Miscarriage, 45, 52, 74, 181, 189,
202-203, 210-211

Moods, 60, 170, 201-203, 205, 207,
209

Morning sickness, 3, 6, 9, 32, 79-83

Motherhood, 203, 214

Motion sickness, 6, 9, 13, 32, 48,
79-82, 186

MSG, 96-97

Multiple births, 66, 184

Multivitamin, 4, 185

Muscles, 6, 24, 67, 77, 160-161,
166, 174, 183, 204

Naps, 175, 223

Nausea, 12, 17, 22, 79, 81-82, 173,
186, 196, 199-200

Nauseous, 186, 188

Neonatal, 78

Nervous, 45, 73, 77

Neural tube disorders, 4, 8, 22

Neurological, 27

Newborn, 67-68

Nicotine, 162, 189

Nipples, 163, 200, 216

Nursing, 63, 66, 164, 198, 204, 215-
217, 220, 224

Nutrients, 5, 7-8, 17, 21-22, 24, 37,
42, 48-49, 60, 67, 73, 96, 98,
104, 106, 135, 165, 167, 185,
189, 193

Nutrition, 3-5, 18, 34, 38, 63-64,
74, 78, 104-105, 121, 172, 185,
190, 195, 227-228, 233

Obesity, 167, 194

Obstetrician, 171

Odors, 81

Omega-3, 27, 215

Osteoporosis, 54, 184

Overuse, 48, 191

Overweight, 65-66, 73-74

Oxygen, 56, 172, 189, 196

Parenthood, 189, 203

Pediatrician, 163, 214, 222

Pelvis, 160-161, 173-174, 191

Period, 5, 66, 78, 81-82, 121, 207,
211, 215, 220

Pesticides, 42

Placenta, 17, 21, 24, 47, 67, 189

Pollution, 52, 172-173, 201

Postpartum, 27, 220, 222-223

Posture, 43, 161

Potassium, 39, 183

Preeclampsia, 171, 194

Premature, 8, 27, 58, 65, 68, 163,
189, 193

Prenatal, 5, 31, 56, 63, 73-74, 81,
183-186, 197, 203, 216

Prepregnancy, 233

Prescription, 3, 44, 56, 59-60, 62,
65, 208

Preservative, 43, 191

BOOKS AND TAPES
BY PAMELA M. SMITH, R.D.

THE GOOD LIFE—A HEALTHY COOKBOOK

A wonderful feast of Pam's most savory recipes. This cookbook offers complete meals for breakfast, lunch, and dinner, plus scrumptious desserts and power-snack ideas. Cooking techniques and plate design are presented in an easy and practical manner, showing that food that is good for you tastes great! For the novice or gourmet cook, this book is designed for everyone to enjoy—and it's beautiful! It's a deluxe hardback edition with full-color photography.

$25.00 each

EAT WELL—LIVE WELL

A BESTSELLER, this is Pam's nutrition guidebook for healthy, productive living. This large, hardback edition presents "The Ten Commandments of Good Nutrition" in detail, along with direction for menu planning, grocery shopping, and dining out—from fast food to gourmet. The large cookbook section contains innovative recipes that can be prepared in a time-saving manner. Meal plans for weight loss and weight management are included.

$20.00 each

THE SEVEN SECRETS TO LIVING THE GOOD LIFE
A VIDEO AND AUDIO TAPE SERIES

In this dynamic four-tape series (audio or video), you will learn how to fit healthy living into your busy schedule, turbo-charge your metabolism and your immune system, seal all the "energy leaks" in your body, and recharge and refuel while you lean down. Pam demonstrates her healthy and delicious cooking techniques and gives easy tips for traveling and dining out healthfully.

4-tape Video Series: $60.00
4-tape Audio Series: $25.00

FOOD FOR LIFE

More than a nutrition guide and cookbook, *Food For Life* shows how to eat smart and walk in abundant life. It presents Pam's secrets for staying fit, fueled, and free—helping you to explore your relationship with food and yourself. You will discover how to choose the best food, manage weight, and develop a proper perspective for feeding yourself emotionally and spiritually. Meal plans, recipes, and specific action steps are included.

Deluxe Hardback Edition: $15.00 each
Paperback Edition: $10.00 each

FOOD FOR LIFE: A-DAY-AT-A-TIME

This thirty-day devotional guide will equip you and empower you to break free of the food trap—forever!

COME COOK WITH ME

This is the kid's cookbook! A wonderful way to teach children nutrition by teaching them the basics of healthy cooking. Great for picky eaters! Includes kid-proven recipes, how to set a table, and some great lessons on manners. Handwritten and fun.

$10.00 each

ALIVE AND WELL IN THE FAST LANE

A lighthearted and informative nutritional guidebook for the whole family—in a fun, handwritten, and illustrated format. Includes tips for healthy eating on the run.

$11.00 each

THE FOOD TRAP SEMINAR—BOOK AND TAPE ALBUM

Hear Pam present a live seminar asking the question, "Is the Refrigerator Light the Light of your Life?" Informative and enlightening, this four-tape audiocassette series and book reveals case studies and personal insights into the physical, emotional, and spiritual aspects of food dependencies. Learn how to break free and live free in all areas of life.

$25.00 each

For more information on
Pamela Smith's books, tapes, speaking,
and seminar/workshops,
please write or call:

Pamela M. Smith, R.D.
P.O. Box 541009
Orlando, FL 32854
800.896.4010 (orders)
407.855.8630 (information)

or

Creation House
600 Rinehart Road
Lake Mary, FL 32746
800.283.8494
800.283.4561 (fax)

Please send Pam your stories and victories at her e-mail address:
PS4Health@aol.com

SPECIAL OFFER
BY PAMELA M. SMITH, R.D.

FREE!

···

"FEEDING YOUR BABY: THE FIRST YEAR"
AUDIOCASETTE TAPE

For a free copy of Pamela Smith's
"Feeding Your Baby: The First Year,"
please complete and mail the following coupon
plus $2.50 (in U.S. currency) to cover postage and handling:

❏ Please send me a free copy of Pamela Smith's "Feeding Your Baby: The First Year" audiocassette tape. I have enclosed $2.50 to cover postage and handling (Canadian residents, please enclose $3.50 U.S. dollars).

❏ Please send me a free Food Diary.

❏ Please send me information on your newsletter.

Name: _____

Address: _____

City: _____ State: _____ Zip: _____

PLEASE SEND COUPON AND CHECK TO:
Pamela M. Smith, R.D.
P.O. Box 541009
Orlando, FL 32854

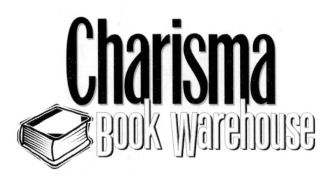
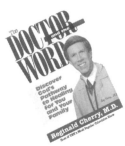
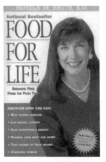
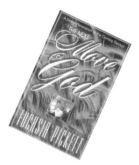

Your Walk With God Can Be Even Deeper ...

With *Charisma* magazine, you'll be informed and inspired by the features and stories about what the Holy Spirit is doing in the lives of believers today.

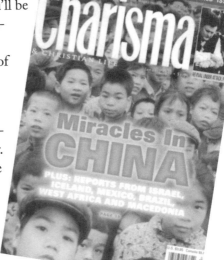

Each issue:

- Brings you exclusive worldwide reports to rejoice over.
- Keeps you informed on the latest news from a Christian perspective.
- Includes miracle-filled testimonies to build your faith.
- Gives you access to relevant teaching and exhortation from the most respected Christian leaders of our day.

Call 1-800-829-3346 for 3 FREE issues
Offer#88ACHB

If you like what you see, then pay the invoice of $21.97 (saving over **$25** OFF the cover price) and receive 9 more issues (12 in all). Otherwise, write "cancel" on the invoice, return it, and owe nothing.

Charisma Offer #88ACHB
P.O. Box 420626
Palm Coast, FL 32142-0626

Experience the Power of Spirit-Led Living